Praise for **Your Nutrition Solution to Acid Reflux**

"Got reflux? Not satisfied with the results you are getting or want to consider alternative treatments? Then this comprehensive resource is a must-read!"

—Jennifer Masters, MS, RD, LDN, CLT

"Guaranteed to give the reader a greater understanding of the underlying causes behind reflux symptoms. Kimberly provides a plethora of practical solutions to not just alleviate the symptoms but to find the individualized treatment to resolve them. Anyone who reads and follows will have relief!"

—Elizabeth Berry, MS, RD, Nutrition Vision, LLC

"Kim takes the complex subject of acid reflux and helps you not only understand the condition and why you are struggling with it, but also leads you through the medical, alternative, and lifestyle solutions to help you find lasting relief. Instead of popping Tums, use Kim's nutrition toolkit to get to the root of your reflux and help you feel better for good!"

—Michaela Ballmann, MS, RD, CLT, dietitian and Functional Nutrition Counselor, Wholify

"**Your Nutrition Solution to Acid Reflux** is an easy-to-read book that everyone who has ever suffered from gastric distress will benefit from. It is factual and full of evidence-based facts stated in terms everyone can understand. I find it well-planned, easy and interesting to read, and simply stated. I plan to recommend this book to my clients as soon as it is published."

—Digna Cassens, MHA, RDN, Diversified Nutrition Management Systems

"**Your Nutrition Solution to Acid Reflux** is packed with all the information one would need to understand the causes and various forms of acid reflux. Also, as a dietitian, I appreciated the detailed nutritional relief suggestions. A good read for anybody."

—Peggy Korody, RD, RD4Health Nutrition Counseling, LLC

"This book delivers evidence-based practice for healthy eating and acid reflux together in an organized and intuitive format. Kim does a beautiful job of walking the reader through the information and providing a vast array of resources. I love the 'Nutrition Solution Tidbits,' as they organize the information into digestible sound bites for easy reference. Good job, Kim! I can't wait to keep this book on my shelf as a reference!"

—Whitney Ahneman, MS, RDN, CLT

"I love this book. It is one of the most comprehensive and well-written books on the subject of reflux and GERD that I have read."

—Sharon Richmond, MBA, RD, LDN, CLT, Nutrition Your Weigh!

your nutrition
SOLUTION
to
ACID REFLUX

your nutrition
SOLUTION
to
ACID REFLUX

a meal-based plan to help manage acid reflux,
heartburn, and other symptoms of GERD

kimberly a. tessmer, RDN, LD

New Page Books
a division of The Career Press, Inc.
Pompton Plains, N.J.

YOUR NUTRITION SOLUTION TO ACID REFLUX
EDITED AND TYPESET BY KARA KUMPEL
Cover design by Joanna Williams
Printed in the U.S.A.

To order this title, please call toll-free 1-800-CAREER-1 (NJ and Canada: 201-848-0310) to order using VISA or MasterCard, or for fur-ther infor-mation on books from Career Press.

The Career Press, Inc.
220 West Parkway, Unit 12
Pompton Plains, NJ 07444
www.careerpress.com
www.newpagebooks.com

Library of Congress Cataloging-in-Publication Data
Tessmer, Kimberly A., author.
    Your nutrition solution to acid reflux : a meal-based plan to help manage acid reflux, heartburn, and other symptoms of GERD / by Kimberly A. Tessmer, RD, LD.
        pages cm
    Includes bibliographical references and index.
    ISBN 978-1-60163-323-1 -- ISBN 978-1-60163-444-3 (ebook) 1. Gastroesophageal reflux--Nutritional aspects. 2. Gastroesophageal reflux--Diet therapy--Recipes. I. Title.

    RC815.7.T47 2014
    616.3'240654--dc23
                                        2014000408

Disclaimer

At the time of writing, all information in this book was believed by the author to be correct and accurate. However, information on acid reflux changes frequently as more research is being completed. Always keep yourself up to date by reading reputable and current publications and speaking with your healthcare provider. The author shall have no liability of any kind for damages of any nature, however caused. The author will not accept any responsibility for any omissions, misinterpretations, or misstatements that may exist within this book. The author does not endorse any product or company listed in this book. Always consult with your healthcare provider for medical advice as well as recommendations on any type of supplement you plan on taking. The author is not engaged in rendering medical services and this book should not be construed as medical advice nor should it take the place of being properly diagnosed and monitored by your regular healthcare provider.

Dedication

I dedicate this book to all of those people out there who deal with acid reflux and GERD every day—including myself. My hope is that this book will help you relieve the frustration that goes along with dealing with acid reflux on a regular basis and empower you to make the necessary changes to start feeling better.

As always, I also dedicate this book to my dad and to my late mom, whom I miss dearly. I am so thankful for the gift they passed on to me for helping others. That is what gives me my passion to be a dietitian and to help others deal with their struggles.

Acknowledgments

I'd like to extend a loving thank-you to my wonderful husband, Greg, who works so hard, which allows me to do what I love, and to my daughter, Tori, who is always patient and gives Mommy the time to do her writing. I would like to thank my fellow RDs who gave me their expert input and advice on this subject. A special thank-you also goes to Susan Linke, MBA, MS, RD, LD, CLT, and Jan Patenaude, RD, CLT, for all of their help with this book.

contents

introduction

Most of us have experienced that uncomfortable, fiery sensation in our chest after we eat a big meal or foods that don't quite agree with us—the dreaded heartburn! The good news is that despite its name it actually has nothing to do with your heart. The "heartburn" sensation you feel is, in medical terms, *acid reflux*. When acid reflux becomes a chronic problem it is called GERD, or *gastroesophageal reflux disease*.

Heartburn caused by acid reflux is a very common problem in the United States. In fact, it is estimated that more than a whopping 15 million Americans suffer with some type of acid reflux, GERD, or other esophageal disorders. Because so many people self-treat themselves at home without even seeing their doctor, the number is probably much higher than we even realize.

Your first step, before even reading this book, is to consult with your doctor (if you haven't already). Make sure the symptoms you are experiencing are actually those of acid reflux or GERD. Once you know that is your problem, you can begin to fix it. Don't fall into the trap of popping over-the-counter pills every time you eat just to relieve your impending symptoms. Now is the time to get to the root of your discomfort. Work with your doctor to develop the best treatment plan for you. The good news is that the majority of heartburn and/or acid reflux issues can be rectified with smart lifestyle changes, including changing the foods and beverages you consume.

If you are not sure where to start, then do I have the book for you! This book will be enlightening for anyone suffering with the discomfort and frustration of acid reflux or GERD. It will provide you with essential information on acid reflux, and, even better, it will take you step by step and provide you with the tools you need to pinpoint your triggers, which will help combat your symptoms and start you living a life free of heartburn. You cannot rely on over-the-counter or prescription medications alone or for a long period of time. Instead, making changes to your nutritional intake and lifestyle habits is the solution you can count on for long-term relief. It is time to take charge of your own health, and this book is your nutrition solution to acid reflux!

chapter 1

your questions about acid reflux—answered

So your doctor has told you that you have acid reflux or maybe even GERD. Now what? What does that mean? Naturally you have loads of important questions swirling around in your head. This chapter provides some common questions and their answers that can help you sort through all of the basic information surrounding acid reflux and GERD. Once you have a better understanding of the *hows*, *whats*, and *whys* of acid reflux, you will be ready to dive into the nutrition and lifestyle changes you need to make you feel better and prevent future damage. This is a perfect starting point!

What Is Acid Reflux?

First of all, if you have been told you have acid reflux, don't feel alone. A good 10 percent of Americans suffer with some degree of heartburn or acid reflux. In fact, it is much more common now than it was in the past. A long-term study found that the number of people who experience acid reflux at least once a week has gone up almost 50 percent in the last 10 years, with women appearing to be a bit more susceptible than men. That may say a little something about our current American diet!

Basically, acid reflux occurs when the liquid content from your stomach, the gastric acid, backs up or "refluxes" into the esophagus. More specifically, at the entrance to your stomach, between the esophagus and the stomach, there is a valve made of muscle called the *lower esophageal sphincter* or LES. When functioning normally the LES closes immediately following food passing through the esophagus and through the valve, keeping the contents of your stomach where it belongs—in your stomach. If the LES is not functioning normally, either by not closing all the way or opening too often, the liquid, which contains stomach acids among other stomach juices, can squeeze through the LES and move back up into the esophagus. This can cause irritation of the lining of the esophagus, resulting in symptoms of burning and chest pain known as *heartburn*.

Are Acid Reflux, Heartburn, and GERD All the Same Problem?

No. Although the terms *acid reflux, heartburn,* and *GERD* are often used interchangeably, they don't all have the same definition. **Acid reflux** is the act of acid from the stomach refluxing back up through the LES and into the esophagus. **Heartburn** is a *symptom* of acid reflux and is the actual burning and pain that one might feel due to acid reflux. **Gastroesophageal Reflux Disease (GERD)** occurs when your symptoms of acid reflux, including heartburn, become chronic and flare up at least twice every week.

> **Your Nutrition Solution Tidbit:** The term gastroesophageal means "relating to the stomach and esophagus." The esophagus is the tube that transports food from your mouth into your stomach.

What Is "Silent" Reflux?

Laryngopharyngeal reflux, or LPR, is often referred to as "silent reflux." Similar to GERD, LPR is also caused by acid reflux. However, the symptoms are usually different from those typically found with GERD. This makes LPR difficult to diagnose, and is why it is sometimes termed "silent" reflux. There are two valves or sphincters at both ends of the esophagus. With LPR both sphincters do not function correctly so that acidy stomach contents reflux back up into the esophagus and keep going all the way through the top valve. This causes stomach acid to back up into places a bit higher such as your throat (pharynx), voice box (larynx), and sometimes even your nasal passages. The result is inflammation in areas that are not equipped to protect against gastric acid.

> **Your Nutrition Solution Tidbit:** The term *laryngopharyngeal* is defined as "pertaining to the larynx (voice box) and the pharynx (throat)."

Silent reflux can be common in infants because (a) the valves of their esophagus are not fully developed, (b) they have a shorter esophagus, and (c) they lie down the majority of the time.

Symptoms in infants and children may include:

- Hoarseness
- "Barking" or chronic cough
- Asthma-like symptoms such as wheezing
- Noisy or irregular breathing
- Chronic spitting-up
- Trouble gaining weight

The symptoms in adults can include heartburn, but other signs are less typical than those found in GERD. Often the symptoms are so vague that they are easily confused with other issues, which makes silent reflux tough to identify and diagnose. In addition to possible heartburn, adults with laryngopharyngeal or silent reflux may experience:

- Bitter taste in the mouth after eating
- Burning sensation in back of throat
- Chronic throat clearing
- Persistent cough
- Mild voice hoarseness
- Sore throat
- The feeling of a lump in the throat that does not go away with repeated swallowing

Other less common symptoms include:

- Postnasal drip or excessive mucus in the throat
- Trouble swallowing
- Trouble breathing

Although silent reflux is a bit harder to diagnose through symptoms alone, your doctor can diagnose the problem through a combination of a medical history and a physical exam. If further testing is needed, an upper endoscopy procedure, barium swallow test, and/or pH test, which measures the level of acid in the throat, may be performed. Once diagnosed, as with acid reflux and GERD, silent reflux should be treated with a combination of diet and lifestyle change and possible medications. Without treatment, silent reflux can cause some long-term damage. The irritation of the stomach acid to the throat and larynx can scar the throat and voice box, cause ulcers on the vocal cords, lead to a chronic cough, and increase your risk for cancer in the affected areas. It can also affect the lungs and aggravate pre-existing conditions such as asthma, emphysema, and/or bronchitis. In infants and children, if left untreated, silent reflux can cause contact ulcers, recurrent ear infections, and possible narrowing of the area below the vocal cords due to a buildup of scar tissue. So, although "silent," laryngopharyngeal reflux is nothing to ignore!

What Are the Signs and Symptoms of Acid Reflux and/or GERD?

The symptoms of acid reflux can be extremely individualized. Some people will experience more symptoms than others, and some will experience more severity and more frequency than others. The most classic symptom of acid reflux and GERD is heartburn. However, did you know that there are a variety of other symptoms associated with acid reflux and GERD? That's right! You may be experiencing other symptoms without even realizing that they are associated with acid reflux. These symptoms can include:

- **Regurgitation.** Regurgitation is the sensation of stomach acid backing up into the back of your throat and sometimes into the mouth. It can cause a bitter taste in the mouth.

- **Dysphagia** (difficulty swallowing). Some people may experience difficulty or pain when swallowing. It may even feel like you have a lump in your throat.

א **Dyspepsia** (stomach discomfort). Some people may experience dyspepsia, which is a general term for stomach discomfort. This might include chronic burping, nausea after eating, stomach fullness and/or bloating, and upper abdominal pain and discomfort after a meal, especially a big one.

א **Pain or a feeling of heartburn when lying down.** When we are seated upright gravity takes over and stomach acid tends to stay where it belongs. When lying down there is more of a tendency for reflux to take over and for the acid to move into the esophagus. This can cause trouble with sleeping.

Other less common signs and symptoms include chronic sore throat, hoarseness, non-burning chest pain, worsening dental issues, chronic cough, wheezing, and even recurrent lung infections.

Your Nutrition Solution Tidbit: Although chest pain can be a symptom of acid reflux and GERD, it can be difficult to tell what is actually causing the chest pain. If you experience chest pain, especially pain that worsens with physical exertion, seek medical attention immediately.

How Is Acid Reflux Diagnosed?

First let's start with the type of doctor you need to visit if you believe you are experiencing symptoms of acid reflux. A *gastroenterologist* is the doctor that specializes in the digestive system and its disorders such as acid reflux and GERD. If you experience classic symptoms of heartburn it may be fairly easy for your doctor to diagnose your issue as acid reflux. If your acid reflux doesn't ease with treatment or you have other troubling symptoms your doctor may order testing to pinpoint any further problems and/or complications. If this is the case your doctor may order one or more of the following tests.

Endoscopy

This procedure is the gold standard in testing where acid reflux and GERD are concerned. It is an outpatient exam that can be used to determine the cause of chronic reflux or GERD as well as silent reflux by providing the doctor with a visual of your upper GI system. Although most people with reflux will have an esophagus that looks normal, an endoscopy can detect esophagitis (inflammation of the lining of the esophagus) as well as erosions and/or ulcers, which can substantiate a diagnosis of GERD. An endoscopy can also identify complications of GERD and/or other problems that might be causing symptoms similar to GERD, such as ulcers, strictures, Barrett's esophagus, and several types of cancers. Your doctor will provide you with pre-testing guidelines that you will need to follow closely.

During this procedure, medication is applied to numb the back of the throat, and a mild sedative is given. The doctor then uses a thin scope with a light and camera at the tip to explore your upper digestive system, which includes the esophagus, stomach, and the upper part of your small intestines, called the duodenum. During the test the doctor may take small tissue samples (biopsy) for further testing of underlying diseases such as esophageal cancer and/or celiac disease. It may sound scary but it only takes 15 to 30 minutes, and before you know it you are back in recovery.

> **Your Nutrition Solution Tidbit:** New technology is emerging regarding endoscopies. Doctors may soon be able to utilize a much easier way of screening the esophagus for conditions such as Barrett's esophagus, esophageal cancer, hiatal hernia, and esophagitis. This new procedure involves simply swallowing a capsule the size of a multivitamin containing optical frequency domain imaging (OFDI), which is tethered to a string-like device. This new procedure will not require patient sedation or specialized equipment. Good news for patients!

Barium Swallow (or Upper GI Series)

This procedure can detect changes to the lining within your esophagus, and may be used to rule out any possible structural problems as well. This test is also outpatient and completely painless. You will be asked to swallow a chalky barium solution that will coat the lining of your digestive tract. A technician will then take X-rays of your esophagus and upper digestive tract. This will allow the doctor, radiologist, and possibly a speech therapist (depending on your individual symptoms) to view the shape and condition of not only your esophagus but your stomach and upper intestine (duodenum) as well. Although this procedure may be used, it is not a gold-standard test for diagnosing GERD. The problem is that very few people with GERD have changes in the lining of the esophagus that would be visible on x-rays, so it could show negative when in fact a patient has GERD. The test can reveal some complications of GERD such as ulcers and strictures, so it is best used along with endoscopy.

Esophageal pH Monitoring

This procedure is used to identify when and for how long stomach acid is found in the esophagus. It has two versions: the more traditional version utilizes an acid-measuring sensor attached to thin, flexible tubing. The tube is threaded through the nose and down into the esophagus so that the sensor ends up in your lower esophagus. The tube is left in place for 24 hours, with the part of the tube that exits your nose wrapped around the ear and trailing down to the waist, where it is connected to a small recording device that is easily worn or carried. During the 24-hour period of testing, you will be asked to record in a diary when you eat and drink. Each time acid reflux occurs into the esophagus, it stimulates the sensor and records the episode. The detailed information that is collected by both you and the sensor will aid the doctor in analyzing and interpreting your test results. Another, newer version of the pH test utilizes a small pH sensor or probe that is affixed to your lower esophagus using suction. The probe is put in place via a tube inserted through the nose or mouth with little to no discomfort. Once the probe is in place the tube is removed. The probe communicates wirelessly with a recording device usually worn on the waist for about 48 hours. Eventually the probe will fall off and will pass through the remainder of the digestive tract. After 48 hours, the information from the recording device is downloaded to a computer so that the doctor can analyze and interpret the information to help diagnose your symptoms.

Both versions of this test yield similar information, but the wireless pH test seems to be much more pleasant and easier to deal with. The pH study is expensive and is not considered a gold standard for testing when it comes to GERD because some people without GERD have abnormal amounts of acid in their esophagus, so a diagnosis of GERD would require further evidence such as typical symptoms, response to treatment, and/or possible complications of GERD. However, the test *can* determine, in patients who do not respond to medication treatment, *why* treatment is ineffective. If the test reveals that there are still substantial amounts of acid in the esophagus while a patient is on prescribed medications, the doctor will assume the treatment is ineffective and needs to be changed. If the test reveals that acid suppression is normal and therefore there is minimal reflux, but the patient is still experiencing symptoms, then the diagnosis of GERD is most likely incorrect, and determining the causes of symptoms will require further testing.

Your Nutrition Solution Tidbit: pH, or potential of hydrogen, is a measurement that reveals whether a solution is acid or alkaline. Gastric fluid that is formed in our stomachs contains hydrochloric acid, which is responsible for the acidic pH value. The acid aides in digestion of the foods and beverages we consume.

Esophageal Motility Testing

This test determines how well the muscles of the esophagus are functioning. For this test, as with some of the others, a thin tube called a catheter is passed through the nose and into the esophagus. The part of the catheter that lies inside the esophagus contains sensors that detect pressure. Pressure within the esophagus is created when the muscles of the esophagus contract. The part of the catheter that comes from the nose is hooked to a monitor that records the pressure. During the test, the contractions of the lower esophageal sphincter are evaluated by having the patient take sips of water. This type of test is used in evaluating symptoms that are not responding to traditional treatment for GERD because abnormal functioning of the esophageal muscle can sometimes mirror the symptoms of GERD. Motility testing can help to identify possible abnormalities and lead to a different diagnosis of esophageal motility disorder.

Gastric Emptying Study

This type of test determines how effectively food is being emptied from the stomach. A small percentage of people with GERD have slow emptying of the stomach that could contribute to the problem of acid reflux. In this test the patient eats a meal with a radioactive substance added. A sensor is placed over the stomach that measures how quickly the radioactive substance in the meal empties from the stomach. This test can be useful for patients with GERD who might not be responding to medication treatment as expected. If the test shows slow gastric emptying the doctor might prescribe additional medication to speed up the emptying of the stomach. In addition, symptoms such as nausea, vomiting, or chronic regurgitation can be the result of either abnormal gastric emptying or GERD. Evaluating gastric emptying therefore can also be useful in identifying patients whose symptoms are due to abnormal emptying of the stomach and not GERD.

What Can Cause Acid Reflux?

People of all ages, from infants whose digestive tracts aren't quite fully developed to the elderly whose digestive systems tend to slow down—and everyone in between—can develop acid reflux. It is difficult to pinpoint exactly what causes acid reflux and GERD, but there are some factors that can make some people more prone to acid reflux:

- Overuse of alcohol
- Obesity
- Smoking (which can substantially reduce the clearance of acid from the esophagus)
- Pregnancy

≈ Certain medications such as calcium channel blockers, medications for asthma, and some anti-histamines, painkillers, and antidepressants

In addition, there are a few medical conditions that can also contribute to problems of acid reflux and GERD. These include hiatal hernias and food allergies/sensitivities.

Hiatal Hernias

A hiatal hernia can occur in people of any age, though it is more common in older adults, even those who are otherwise healthy. A good majority of people—though not all—who have GERD also have a hiatal hernia, but a hiatal hernia is not always the cause of GERD. A hiatal hernia occurs when a small portion of the upper stomach moves up into the chest area above the diaphragm, which is the muscle that separates the stomach from the chest. The diaphragm normally helps the (lower esophagus sphincter) LES keep gastric acid from coming up into the esophagus from the stomach by contracting. In the case where a hiatal hernia is present, there is a weakening in the diaphragm muscle at the hiatus, allowing the stomach to partially slip through the diaphragm into the chest. This makes it easier for acid to flow back up, making acid reflux more likely. Some people who have hiatal hernias do not experience symptoms of acid reflux. For these people, their hiatal hernia produces no symptoms. The exact cause of hiatal hernias is at present unknown, but the loosening of the tissue that surrounds the diaphragm that can occur with age can be one culprit. There is no way to prevent hiatal hernias.

Food Allergies/Reactions

Research has concluded that food sensitivities and allergies play a role in many common health conditions, including GERD. Essentially, your symptoms of acid reflux can be caused by your immune system's reaction to a certain food, additive, or other substance in your diet. Sometimes it can be a food or beverage that is easy to identify, such as milk. Other times it can be a chemical or a food additive, which can be extremely difficult to identify. *Any* food or food additive can be reactive in a person. Even foods such as chicken or garlic can cause symptoms. Sometimes these reactions can be delayed and/or can depend on the amount you have consumed. This means you may not feel the effects of the reaction for hours or days after eating the reactive food, or until you've eaten enough of the food. This can make trying to identify the offending food very difficult. Mediator Release Testing (MRT) is a patented blood test that quantifies how strongly your immune cells react to certain foods and food chemicals. Chapter 3 will discuss more about testing for reactive foods.

Can H. pylori Cause Acid Reflux?

H. pylori, which is short for Helicobacter pylori, is a bacteria often found in the stomach that is able to penetrate the protective mucous lining of the stomach, where it produces substances that weaken the lining and make the stomach more susceptible to damage caused by gastric acids, such as peptic ulcers and gastritis. Over time, H. pylori can increase one's risk for stomach cancer. Having H. py-lori doesn't guarantee that you will end up with ulcers or stomach cancer, but it can increase the odds. The good news is that most people who become infected with the bacteria never even experience symptoms or problems. Only a small percentage of people develop stomach cancer, and it is not clear why some people with the bacteria develop ulcers and others don't. If people do have symptoms, they are usually symptoms of gastritis or peptic ulcers, with the most common symptoms being burning and pain in the stomach, just beneath the ribs. Symptoms tend to improve when you eat food, drink milk, or take an antacid, and worsen if your stomach is empty. People may also experience symptoms of weight loss, loss of appetite, bloating, burping, and nausea. H. pylori is diagnosed by tests such as an upper GI series, endoscopy, blood test, and/or stool test. It is normally treated with antibiotics, medications such as H2 blockers and proton-pump inhibitors (PPIs) to reduce possible stomach acid, and, if needed, ulcer surgery. Doctors normally recommend the same type of diet for H. pylori as for acid reflux, advising patients to avoid spicy, fatty, and acidic foods.

Now that you know what H. pylori is, the answer to whether it can cause acid reflux is no. And at this point experts believe that this bacteria does not cause GERD. Some studies actually suggest that H. pylori may have a protective effect against GERD by reducing stomach acid. Studies have shown that patients who are treated for H. pylori can develop symptoms of GERD once the bacteria have been killed off with treatment.

Because some of the symptoms of GERD and H. pylori bacteria can mirror each other, if you present to your doctor with certain symptoms he or she most likely will do an endoscopy and check for H. pylori to ensure that isn't the problem. Some people who have H. pylori with existing GERD and who are taking acid-reducing medications can end up with issues in the stomach. Scientists are not quite sure how people end up with the H. pylori infection but at this time believe it may be contracted through food and water.

Can Too Little Stomach Acid Cause Acid Reflux or GERD?

We have talked quite a bit about stomach or gastric acid, and so far it probably sounds like something evil. But the fact is, acid in the stomach is essential to proper digestion of foods and beverages. Our stomachs are devised in such a way that they are protected from their own acidic properties. In the case of acid reflux, it is not that your stomach is producing too much acid, but that improper functioning of the lower esophageal sphincter or valve allows the stomach acid to escape up into the esophagus.

Because of the functions acid serves during digestion, numerous problems can occur when stomach acid is too low. For example, nutrients from the foods we consume cannot be broken down properly, especially proteins, so they tend to sit in the stomach and take way too long to digest, which causes reflux. In addition, low stomach acid promotes an environment that is more receptive to the growth of microorganisms that are fed by the carbohydrates that sit in the stomach too long, again because of low acidity. This eventually results in excessive pressure within the stomach from the bacterial overgrowth and the not-quite-digested food.

The stomach has two valves, one we talked about, the LES, which sits at the top of the stomach and connects to the esophagus. That valve is designed to open both ways, meaning liquids can go through both ways. The other valve sits at the bottom of the stomach and is called the pyloric sphincter. That valve is a one-way route that allows digested material to enter the small intestines. When the stomach experiences low acid and the buildup of pressure we spoke about earlier, and the gastric juices are not at the acidic level they need to be at to allow for the opening of the pyloric sphincter, the body is smart enough to know there is only one way out to relieve the pressure: back through the LES and into the esophagus, which in turn can cause acid reflux and the feeling of heartburn. So even though this is being caused by too little acid, there will still be enough acid in those gastric juices that flow back up into the esophagus to cause symptoms of heartburn. If this begins to happen frequently, eventually it will contribute to a weakened LES, which compounds the problem and can result in GERD. This is often an overlooked issue when it comes to diagnosing acid reflux and GERD.

There are a whole host of other health problems that can occur from low stomach acid. People who have been diagnosed with other gastrointestinal issues are usually at higher risk for lower stomach acid. Some symptoms could include not feeling well after eating meat, excessive burping or gas after meals, as well as extensive stomach bloating and/or heartburn after meals. Because so many of these symptoms mirror other issues it is difficult to diagnose by symptoms alone. If you have made the necessary diet and lifestyle changes and are still suffering with acid reflux you may want to speak with your doctor about the possibility of low stomach acid levels as a probable cause.

How Can I Find Out if I Have Low Stomach Acid?

Here are some tests that can be used to test for low stomach acid.

The Heidelberg Stomach Acid Test

This gold standard test is more costly than others you can do, but it will give you the best results. This test needs to be done in your doctor's office. The Heidelberg test works by using a small capsule, the size of a vitamin, equipped with a radio transmitter. The transmitter records the pH of your stomach (the acidity versus alkalinity) as you drink a solution of sodium bicarbonate (baking soda) to neutralize the hydrochloric acid in the stomach. You are asked to fast for eight to 12 hours overnight before the test and take no acid-suppressing medications for at least four days prior to the test. You then swallow the pill-sized capsule and drink the solution. The test will continuously record the pH in your stomach for as long as needed until there are definitive results. The results of the test show up on a graph that reveals your pH levels at regular intervals of time, allowing your doctor to diagnose whether you consistently have low stomach acid even after neutralizing your stomach acid with the baking soda solution. After the test is finished they will most likely allow the capsule to pass through the intestines and be expelled naturally. This test can be used for other stomach-related acid issues as well.

The Baking Soda Stomach Acid Test

This test can be done at home, for the price of a box of baking soda. However, it is not scientifically proven and will probably not be 100-percent accurate. For this test you drink a baking soda (sodium bicarbonate) solution that creates a chemical reaction in your stomach between the baking soda and your stomach acid or hydrochloric acid (HCL). This combination results in the production of carbon dioxide gas, which causes you to burp. There are a lot of variables to control, so it is recommended to perform the test for at least three consecutive mornings to find an average and to look for more of a pattern then a yes-or-no answer.

To take this test, mix a quarter-teaspoon of baking soda with about 8 ounces of cold water (make sure it is completely dissolved) and drink the solution first thing in the morning, before anything else goes in your mouth. Time how long it takes you to burp once you drink it. If you do not burp within five minutes it may be a sign of low stomach acid. It is assumed that if your stomach is producing enough acid you should burp within two to three minutes. If you start burping right away and repeatedly it may be a sign that you have too much stomach acid. Be careful not to confuse actual belching with small little burps from swallowing air when you drink the concoction. Because the time frames can vary so much from one individual to another, as well as how fast or slow you drink the solution, this test is only a good indicator that you may need to speak with your doctor about further testing. This type of test, though simple and inexpensive, is not accurate enough to completely rule out or diagnose low stomach acid.

Betaine HCL Challenge Test

The Betaine HCL challenge test is another test you can perform at home, but it is much more reliable than others. You don't need a special kit, which some Websites will try selling you; all you need to purchase is a supplement called *Betaine HCL with Pepsin* (650 mg or less per pill). Next, eat a high-protein meal that includes at least 6 ounces of a lean meat such as steak, poultry, or fish. In the middle of your meal take one Betaine HCL pill. Finish your meal and then pay attention to your body. If you feel basically nothing, you may have low stomach acid. If you start to feel stomach distress such as bloating, heaviness, burning, and so on, then you most likely do not have low stomach acid and may be overproducing stomach acid. As with other at-home tests, this test is not 100-percent fool-proof. You should repeat the test a few times to confirm any results. One of the biggest problems with skewed results is the amount of protein you eat, so be sure to eat enough. After getting at least two positive test results speak with your doctor about the possibility of low stomach acid as the cause of your acid reflux.

> **Your Nutrition Solution Tidbit: Warning:** If you take NSAIDs (nonsteroidal anti-inflammatory drugs) such as aspirin, Motrin, Aleve, or Celebrex, or corticosteroids on a regular basis, the combination with Betaine HCL can increase your risk for gastritis, so speak with your doctor before trying this test or using this supplement.

How Will My Acid Reflux be Treated?

Once you have been properly diagnosed with acid reflux or GERD the next obvious question is, *How will it be treated?* I will touch on it just in general here, as the remainder of the book will delve into this topic in much more detail, especially the nutrition element.

There are varying degrees of acid reflux and GERD, so treatment will be individualized depending on your specific case, but lifestyle changes are always a good first step, including weight loss if necessary, eating smaller meals, and avoiding foods that trigger *your* heartburn symptoms. Some people suffer mostly at night and can find relief by avoiding large meals before bedtime and raising the head of the bed slightly. Giving up smoking, if you are a smoker, can be a big change, as smoking can be a major trigger for acid reflux by weakening the valve in your upper esophagus. There are also medications, both prescription and over-the-counter, that can be used in the short term to help treat the damage and lessen the symptoms that acid reflux can cause. However, keep in mind that medications will only treat the symptoms, such as heartburn, and not the cause of your acid reflux. Lifestyle changes most definitely need to be a larger part of your treatment plan. The most important point here is that acid reflux *needs to be treated!* If left untreated it can cause irritation of the esophagus that can lead to bleeding, ulcers, and scarring as well as more serious health issues such as cancer.

What Type of Medication Is Used to Treat Acid Reflux?

A variety of both over-the-counter and prescription medications are used to treat the symptoms of acid reflux and GERD. Always be properly diagnosed before using any type of medication, even if it is over-the-counter. Masking symptoms, without knowing the true cause, can cause more problems down the line. Each of these medications have pros and cons to taking them, especially long-term.

Antacids

Antacids such as TUMS, Rolaids, and Mylanta are usually a first-line approach to help relieve the symptoms of acid reflux and GERD. They are fast-acting and work by neutralizing the acid in the stomach so that there is no acid to reflux into the esophagus. The problem is that their action is brief and they are emptied from the stomach pretty quickly, allowing for more acid to then re-accumulate. The most effective way to take antacids is about one hour after a meal so that they are working just before the symptoms of reflux would begin. Because consuming food slows stomach emptying, taking an antacid after meals allows it to stay in the stomach longer and therefore be more effective.

Antacids can be aluminum-, magnesium-, or calcium-based. Calcium-based products are unlike other antacids because they stimulate the release of gastrin from the stomach and duodenum. Gastrin is a hormone that is responsible for the stimulation of acid production by the stomach. This causes the production of acid to rebound quicker after the direct acid-neutralizing effect of the calcium carbonate wears off. Therefore, this might not be the best choice for GERD patients. Treatment with antacids containing calcium carbonate has not been shown to be less effective or less safe than treatment with other types of antacids, but in theory calcium-containing antacids are not recommended for frequent use. The occasional use of these products is not believed to be harmful. They do have the advantage, at a low cost, of adding calcium to the diet.

As far as other types of antacids, aluminum-containing products have a tendency to cause constipation, and magnesium-containing antacids tend to cause diarrhea for some people. If this becomes an issue you want to discontinue use and switch to something else. Antacids should only be used occasionally and on a short-term basis while you and your doctor are trying to pinpoint your trigger foods and make necessary lifestyle changes.

> **Your Nutrition Solution Tidbit**: Always follow label instructions on any medication, whether it is over-the-counter or prescription. Taking more than what is directed can sometimes have serious side effects even if it is an over-the-counter medication. If what you are taking is not working, contact your doctor.

H2 Blockers or H2RAs (Histamine Type 2 Antagonists)

Histamine is a chemical that stimulates the production of acid in the stomach. These types of medications, such as cimetidine (Tagamet), famotidine (Pepcid), nizatidine (Axid), and ranitidine (Zantac), work to decrease acid production by blocking the receptor for histamine, therefore preventing histamine from stimulating the acid-producing cells. Because histamine works to stimulate acid after food is consumed, H2RAs are best taken 30 minutes before you eat a meal. This way the medication will be at peak levels in your body when your stomach is at its most active in producing acid. These medications can also be used before bedtime to help suppress nighttime production of gastric acids. These types of medications are used primarily to relieve symptoms of heartburn related to GERD rather than for the healing of esophagitis that may accompany GERD.

These medications were once strictly prescription but are now available both over the counter and with a prescription, depending on strength. Your doctor may prescribe antacids along with these to help control your symptoms. H2RAs work for a longer period of time than antacids but they are not as fast-acting.

PPIs (Proton Pump Inhibitors)

Another type of medication available specifically for acid-related diseases such as GERD is a proton pump inhibitor, or PPI. A PPI blocks the action of acid-secreting cells in the stomach. PPIs tend to shut off acid production more completely and over a longer period of time than H2RAs. PPIs are not only able to treat the symptom of heartburn but can also protect the esophagus from acid so that esophageal inflammation or esophagitis can heal. Doctors usually prescribe PPIs when H2RAs are not successful in relieving symptoms of GERD or when complications such as ulcers, strictures, or Barrett's esophagus exist.

Currently there are six different PPIs that are approved and available for treatment in GERD. Although they are similar in the way they work, they differ in how they are broken down by the liver and how they interact with other medications. The effects of some PPIs last longer than others and can be taken less frequently. PPIs include omeprazole (Prilosec), lansoprazole (Prevacid), rabeprazole (AcipHex), pantoprazole (Protonix), esomeprazole (Nexium), and dexlansorprazole (Dexilant). A seventh type of PPI consists of a combination of omeprazole and sodium bicarbonate (Zegerid). Sodium bicarbonate is an antacid that reduces stomach acid and helps the omeprazole to work more efficiently. Some of these medications can be found in over-the-counter strength as well as prescription strength, whereas others are prescription-strength only. The most-often suggested way of taking PPIs is at least 30 minutes before your first meal of the day. This way you are taking them before you eat, which allows the medication to be at peak level in the body when the stomach is most actively producing acid.

Your Nutrition Solution Tidbit: Esophagitis is inflammation and/or irritation of the esophagus usually caused by GERD.

Prokinetics

Prokinetics are also referred to as pro-motility drugs. They work by stimulating the muscles of the gastrointestinal tract, which includes the esophagus, stomach, small intestines, and colon. Two pro-motility drugs exist: bethanechol (Urecholine) and metoclopramide (Reglan), with Reglan being approved for the treatment of GERD. Although these medications can help to strengthen the lower esophageal sphincter muscle, it is assumed that it is the action of metoclopramide to speed up the emptying of the stomach that is expected to help reduce acid reflux, as it helps shorten the time in which reflux can occur. These types of drugs are most effective if taken 30 minutes before a meal and again at bedtime. Pro-motility drugs are not as effective in treating either the symptoms and/or complications of GERD as other medications have proven to be. Therefore, they are usually reserved for patients who do not respond to other treatments, or are used in conjunction with other treatments for GERD.

Foam Barriers

One more type of medication that can be used as a unique form of treatment for GERD is a foam barrier. There is only one at this time: Gaviscon, which is a combination of aluminum hydroxide gel, magnesium trisilicate, and alginate. Gaviscon is a tablet composed of an antacid and a foaming agent. When the tablet reaches the stomach it disintegrates and then turns into a foam that floats on top of the gastric liquid contents in the stomach. The foam acts as a physical barrier to the reflux of liquid, and the antacid that is bound to the foam neutralizes any acid that comes in contact with the foam. This medication is best taken after meals and when lying down, as these are periods in which reflux is likely to occur. Foam barriers are not used as a first line of treatment, nor are they used as an only form of treatment for GERD. Mainly they are used in combination with other GERD medications when other drugs are not adequately effective in relieving symptoms.

Can I Treat My Acid Reflux With Natural Remedies?

As we mentioned before, reflux can be a very individualized condition. There are many "natural" and alternative treatments, including herbal remedies available. Check out Chapter 2 for more information on this topic.

Can I Treat My Acid Reflux With Medication Alone?

The answer is a resounding NO! Medication, whether over-the-counter or prescription, will basically do two things: First, it may heal the esophagus, if you have inflammation and esophagitis, which is important because that can lead to further complications if not treated. Second, medications will help to control symptoms of GERD such as heartburn. The problem is that you are never getting to the root of the problem or the cause of your acid reflux issues. Taking these medications will become a lifelong situation if you don't dig to find out what factors are causing your problem, and then fix them. Taking medications that treat GERD long-term is not always the answer for everyone and can have health consequences down the line. For the majority of people with acid reflux and GERD the root of the problem is related to nutritional intake and lifestyle. These are factors that you have control of and can make changes to! That is what this book is about: taking control of your health issue and putting the work in to control it instead of continuing your present lifestyle and habits and relying on medications. So, this might not be the answer you were hoping for, but for most people medications alone are not the answer.

Are There Any Complications of GERD that I Should Know About?

Unfortunately there can be possible complications, some serious, of acid reflux and GERD, especially if not properly controlled and left untreated. This is the reason it is so important not to ignore your symptoms of acid reflux. If you experience symptoms you need to see your doctor so that you can start taking action to relieve them and the damage they may be causing.

Esophagitis

As gastric acids repeatedly come into contact with the lining of the esophagus, as happens with acid reflux and GERD, in time it can begin to damage that lining. This damage can cause inflammation, erosions, or ulcers of the lining of the esophagus, which is known as esophagitis. Esophagitis can be painful and cause symptoms such as heartburn, chest pain, difficulty swallowing, and bleeding. Esophagitis is diagnosed with the same type of tests that are used to identify acid reflux. Acid reflux and GERD are just one ailment that can cause esophagitis. Others can include hiatal hernia, medications, infections, food allergies, and radiation therapy. If it has been determined that acid reflux is causing your esophagitis, then treatment would be similar to that for acid reflux.

Strictures

Once the lining of the esophagus becomes damaged by acid reflux and/or esophagitis, it can leave scarring. These scars can cause a narrowing of the esophagus called a *stricture*. Strictures, depending on their severity, can interfere with the swallowing of foods and liquids. Strictures can be treated with dilation, in which a small instrument is placed in the esophagus that gently stretches and expands the opening of the esophagus.

Barrett's Esophagus

Damage to the lining of the esophagus from acid reflux can cause abnormal changes in the lining of the esophagus. This can lead to damage of the cells inside the esophageal lining. In a person with Barrett's esophagus, the normal cells that usually line the esophagus are replaced with a type of cell that is not usually found in that area. Symptoms of this condition mirror those of GERD, and a few people actually experience no symptoms at all. Barrett's esophagus is diagnosed with an upper endoscopy to view the lining of the esophagus and to obtain a biopsy so that a sample of tissue can be examined. Most gastroenterologists recommend an endoscopy to check for Barrett's esophagus in people who have risk factors such as long-term acid reflux and GERD. Treatment goals for Barrett's esophagus include stopping acid reflux to prevent further damage to the lining. Treatment usually includes medications used for acid reflux and GERD as well as lifestyle changes. Some people may require surgery to tighten the sphincter between the esophagus and the stomach to help prevent reflux. The abnormal cells found in Barrett's esophagus can lead to esophageal cancer in about 1 percent of people with GERD each year. Though the risk is low it is still vital that Barrett's esophagus be diagnosed and treated effectively and that people who have been diagnosed undergo regular endoscopies to monitor any changes. For those patients who are at higher risk for developing esophageal cancer, more invasive treatments may be used, such as laser therapy, to destroy the abnormal tissue.

The exact cause of Barrett's esophagus is presently unknown, but GERD has been shown to be a major risk factor for this serious condition. However, people without GERD can also develop Barrett's esophagus. People who have suffered with acid reflux and/or GERD for years may be at higher risk for Barrett's esophagus, though the percentage is low: only about 10 percent of people who have long-term GERD develop this condition. It is typically diagnosed in people of middle age or older, and tends to occur more often in men than in women.

Esophageal Cancer

Esophageal cancer is a type of cancer found in the tissue that lines the esophagus. This type of cancer tends to be more common in men and in people over 65 years of age. Risk factors for cancer of the esophagus include GERD, Barrett's esophagus, cigarette smoking, and drinking alcohol—and especially a combination of any of these.

Cancer that begins in the esophagus is divided into two main types:

1. **Squamous cell carcinoma.** This type of cancer develops in the squamous cells that line the esophagus. It can basically affect any part of the esophagus but tends to be found in the upper and middle areas.

2. **Adenocarcinoma.** This type of cancer develops in gland cells and tends to be found in the lower area of the esophagus. Normally gland cells are not found in the esophagus. When they are found there it is usually due to GERD or Barrett's esophagus.

Cancer of the esophagus, in the early stages, often presents with no symptoms. Generally, difficulty in swallowing is one of the most common symptoms to initially appear, along with weight loss. As the cancer grows, it begins to narrow the opening of the esophagus, making swallowing very difficult and painful.

chapter 2

the nutrition connection and beyond

Now that you have a better understanding of exactly what heartburn, acid reflux, and GERD are, we can take a further look into treating this health issue. This chapter will discuss the treatment of a more delicate population: that of children and pregnant women. You will find out why relying solely on over-the-counter or prescription medications for treatment can be problematic in the long term. Most importantly, this chapter will delve into alternative treatments and supplements that are safe and can be helpful in your fight against acid reflux.

Acid Reflux During Pregnancy

Experiencing acid reflux or GERD during pregnancy is common, even if you didn't have it before you became pregnant. For most it tends to rear its ugly head during the second and third trimesters, and will tend to come and go until your baby is born. It is generally harmless, though it can be uncomfortable; some women will experience worse cases than others.

Symptoms

Symptoms of acid reflux in pregnancy are similar to those in non-pregnancy, with heartburn being the major problem. The only difference is that many women never experience heartburn until they become pregnant, and then once the baby is born their symptoms improve or disappear.

Causes

Heartburn can be a common symptom in pregancy because of changing hormone levels and physical changes in the body that can affect the muscles of the digestive tract and how certain foods are tolerated. During pregnancy, the placenta produces the hormone progesterone, which is intended to relax the muscles of the uterus. However, this hormone also tends to cause the lower esophageal sphincter (LES) to become more relaxed, allowing gastric acids to splash back up into the esophagus, causing acid reflux. In addition, a growing baby can cause an increase in intra-abdominal pressure, which can result in an increase in the development of acid reflux.

Treatment

Treating heartburn during pregnancy can be a bit tricky. Care must be taken when it comes to medications to ensure they are safe for both mom and baby. Your first step is to speak with your healthcare provider concerning your symptoms. The best and safest line of defense is to make dietary and lifestyle changes where possible to help relieve your symptoms. Follow some of the suggestions explained in Step 1 of Chapter 3 regarding eating and lifestyle habits, and follow the Do's and Don'ts of foods in Chapter 4. Gain a sensible amount of weight with your pregnancy and aim to stay within the guidelines your healthcare provider suggests.

If your heartburn persists, speak with your healthcare provider. At that point he or she may prescribe medications that are safe to take during pregnancy. Keep in mind that not all medications are safe during pregnancy, whether over-the-counter or prescription, so refrain from taking anything until you speak with your healthcare provider. In general, antacids such as Mylanta or Maalox can be effective and are safe to take as they are not absorbed into the bloodstream. You might find that the liquid form of these antacids are more effective in controlling your symptoms because they help to coat the esophagus. In addition, chewable and liquid antacids tend to work much quicker than tablets because they are already dissolved. Even though the chewable tablets can be fruity and tasty, if you find yourself popping them too often and in larger quanti-ties than what is recommended, you may need something a bit stronger, such as an H2 blocker. H2 blockers, which we discussed in Chapter 1, such as Zantac, Pepcid, and Tagamet, are absorbed into the bloodstream, but research has not revealed any adverse effects on a developing fe-tus. PPIs such as Nexium, AcipHex, and Prevacid should only be used in severe cases when antacids or H2 blockers are not effective. Research is progressing all the time, so be sure to ask your healthcare provider about potential risks and benefits of taking any of these drugs during preg-nancy. Opt for dietary and lifestyle changes first and use medication only if and when needed.

Your Nutrition Solution Tidbit: Avoid brands of over-the-counter antacids that contain alu-minum (such as aluminum hydroxide or alumi-num carbonate). Aluminum tends to be consti-pating and in large doses can be toxic. So even though they are safe when used occasionally and at the recommended dosage, they are not the best choice during pregnancy. Over-the-counter remedies that contain aspirin should also be avoided during pregnancy. Be aware that aspirin can be listed as salicylate or acetyl-salicylic acid. Steer clear of sodium bicarbon-ate (baking soda), which is sold as an antacid in tablet form, and sodium citrate. Both are high in sodium and can cause unwanted water retention. Always check with your healthcare provider before taking any of these.

Acid Reflux in Infants, Children, and Adolescents

Adults are not the only ones who can suffer from acid reflux. Children and even infants are at risk for what is termed *pediatric* GERD. According to some estimates, between 8 and 25 percent of American children experience frequent symptoms of acid reflux. More than half of infants will experience acid reflux within the first three months of life. For infants, GERD is a more serious form of spitting up and can be quite common. For children and adolescents, GERD is usually diagnosed if they show symptoms more than twice per week and/or experience other complications such as respiratory problems, difficulty gaining weight, and esophagitis.

Symptoms of Pediatric GERD

Signs and symptoms of pediatric GERD can vary greatly depending on age. Symptoms are much more serious than the occasional tummy ache or sporadic spitting-up.

Infants and preschool children may experience:

- Arching of the back during feedings
- Fussiness or irritability, especially while feeding or soon after

- ✂ Refusal to eat or finding it unpleasant
- ✂ Poor weight gain or failure to thrive
- ✂ Weight loss
- ✂ Complaining more than twice per week about a stomach ache or abdominal pain
- ✂ Often complaining of feeling something in the throat or a sore throat
- ✂ Development of breathing problems and/or wheezing
- ✂ Frequent gagging or choking with feeding
- ✂ Excessive hiccups
- ✂ Frequent coughing

Older children and adolescents may experience:

- ✂ Pain or burning in the upper chest (heartburn)
- ✂ Frequent abdominal pain
- ✂ Discomfort or pain when swallowing
- ✂ Chronic coughing, wheezing, or hoarseness
- ✂ Frequent burping
- ✂ Poor weight gain, or weight loss
- ✂ Frequent nausea and/or vomiting
- ✂ A bitter taste or acidic taste in the throat or back of mouth
- ✂ Frequently complaining of a sore throat
- ✂ Feeling that foods gets stuck in the throat
- ✂ Pain that seems to worsen when lying down
- ✂ Recurrent respiratory infections and/or sinusitis

Causes of Pediatric GERD

Although researchers are not exactly sure what always causes GERD in infants and children, there are several factors that may be involved. In infants particularly, the LES has not matured yet, and as a result it isn't able to control acid backup as well as it should. As children get older this should remedy itself. With adolescents and children, genetics may play a role; if a parent suffers from it, his or her child may also. Weight can also be a risk factor, with moderately obese children and adolescents being 30 percent more likely to experience GERD. Overeating can also attribute to GERD. In addition, as with adults, some children my have weak valves that are particularly sensitive to certain foods and beverages (or triggers) that can cause acid reflux.

Treatment for Pediatric GERD

Treatment for pediatric GERD in older children and teens is similar to that for adults, and depends on the severity of the condition. Healthcare providers will almost always advise parents to start their children with diet and lifestyle changes first, such as:

- Eating smaller meals
- Avoiding eating two to three hours before bedtime
- Avoiding carbonated beverages
- Avoiding caffeine
- Avoiding tight-fitting clothes

- Avoiding eating large meals before vigorous activities such as playing sports, and also during times of stress
- Keeping a food diary to look for patterns of foods and beverages that may worsen symptoms
- Regular exercise
- Elevating the head during sleep
- Sleeping on one's left side

See Chapter 3 and Chapter 4 for more tips.

Tips for infants will be different

- Hold the baby upright while feeding.
- Do not lie the baby down for at least 30 to 60 minutes after each feeding
- Elevate the head of the bassinet or crib
- Try smaller feedings more often
- Talk to your doctor about adding solid food if your baby is an older infant
- Talk to your doctor about adding rice cereal to your baby's bottle
- Burp formula-fed infants after they have consumed 1 to 2 oz. of formula; burp breastfed infants after feeding on each side
- If formula feeding, your doctor may recommend changing to a specific type of formula such as a soy formula in case allergies or sensitivities are suspected

If lifestyle and diet changes don't help the child to minimize their symptoms, your doctor may recommend medications in addition to those changes. They can include the same ones we have discussed, including antacids, H2 blockers, and PPIs. There is much debate about starting young children and even infants on these types of medications, especially because not all long-term effects are known, and some that are known are not the best choice for children. It is also not clear whether or not decreasing stomach acid in infants will help to improve reflux. In addition to more serious long-term side effects, some of these medications, whether over-the-counter or prescription, can cause diarrhea or constipation. Refrain from self-treating your child with over-the-counter medications without your doctor's approval. If you are concerned about these issues, speak with your pediatrician and consider trying natural remedies in addition to diet and lifestyle changes instead. Ginger tea, manuka honey (honey should not be given to children younger than 1 year of age), and aloe vera juice are just a few natural remedies that may help relieve the symptoms of pediatric GERD. Your pediatrician may refer your child to a pediatric gastroenterologist if they suspect acid reflux and/or GERD for a more proper diagnosis and treatment plan.

Questioning Medications to Treat GERD Long-term

So, you have been diagnosed with GERD. You figure, *No problem! There are medications to take care of that!* In fact, acid-suppressing medications are the second-highest-selling drugs in the world! So yes, there are medications, which we have previously discussed, that are meant to help relieve your symptoms. These medications will also help to heal possible irritation and inflammation of the esophagus that has occurred due to acid reflux. But—and there is always a "but"—there can be drawbacks to using these medications long-term. Although the long-term safety profile of these types of medications has been proven to be generally good, research has identified a number of problems. You need to understand these drawbacks so that you can speak with your doctor about the pros and cons and decide what is best for you.

Many of these medications have short-term side effects such as diarrhea and constipation, but those usually subside. It is the long-term side effects that become the problem. The general objective of these medications is to suppress the production of stomach acid so that when reflux occurs there isn't as much acid traveling into the esophagus and causing heartburn. The problem with this is that, as we mentioned previously, we actually need acid in our stomach; it is produced there for a reason. Without enough stomach acid, foods are not broken down as effectively, and as a result there is a decrease in the absorption of numerous vitamins and minerals, including calcium, vitamin D, magnesium, B12, and iron. In the long term this can cause osteoporosis, anemia, and other health issues. In addition, there is concern about developing infections because the acid in our stomach helps to kill off the bacteria we swallow. Without the acid production, bacteria may get through to the rest of our body and cause infection, especially in the elderly. For this population these medications can even increase the risk of developing pneumonia. These acid-reducing medications can possibly reduce the effect of other much-needed prescription medications as well. In recent years the Food and Drug Administration (FDA) has issued several warnings concerning PPIs, cautioning people about the long-term use and high doses. A recent warning recommended that older adults use the drugs only for the shortest duration possible. Many people are already deficient in vitamin D and since GERD medications can increase that deficiency, it is important to have your vitamin D levels checked and continue to do that annually. Vitamin D deficiency can increase your risk for a large number of health issues and it can be difficult to get the amount you need through diet and sunlight alone.

Using these drugs for GERD for short periods may not be harmful, but they tend to cause dependency in people, leading them to be used for much longer periods then warranted. Most should only be used for up to six months, but are often used and prescribed for much longer periods of time. When people take these drugs, such as PPIs, and feel relief from their symptoms, they tend to skip the most important part—getting to the root of their problem and making the necessary changes for long-term relief. The big issue here is that eliminating your symptoms will not necessarily protect you from the long-term complications of GERD unless you get to the root of your problem. Some people may need these medications short-term to heal esophagitis or ulcers, and taking them short-term while making diet and lifestyle changes might be helpful, but they are not a long-term solution. Let's not forget price as well. It is much cheaper and better for your overall health in so many ways to permanently change your diet and lifestyle instead. These medications, whether prescription, over-the-counter, or generic, can be quite pricey, especially if taking them on a long-term basis.

So what can you do? First of all, you can visit a registered dietitian nutritionist (RDN) to help you permanently change your diet and nutrition intake for the better. You can try all of the lifestyle and eating habit changes I will discuss later in the book, and lose weight if you are not already at a healthy weight. You can use this book to help you get to the root of your problem and identify your trigger foods so you can knock out the things that are causing you to suffer. You can look into alternative treatments as well. If you must take medication, know that research says prescription and over-the-counter strength H2 blockers and PPIs seem to work equally well to prevent heartburn symptoms and allow the esophagus to heal. In some cases, taking a small dose, especially of a PPI, may work just as well as a large dose. So talk to your doctor, and if your GERD is bad and medication is necessary, ask about taking the lowest dose you can take to at least get your esophagus healed, and ask how long you will need to take it.

Your Nutrition Solution Tidbit: Research has found that people who are overweight do not respond to medications as well. In addition, that extra weight can be the culprit of your GERD in the first place. If weight is an issue, one of your first lines of defense should be to try to reduce your weight in a healthy manner.

Alternative Treatments

There are other ways to treat GERD that can be very helpful along with diet and lifestyle changes. Not all are scientifically proven to help yet, but research continues, and in the meantime they can give you an alternative to medications. Alternative and/or natural treatments are not for everyone, so speak with your doctor first before making any changes to medications or adding any type of natural or herbal supplement.

Your Nutrition Solution Tidbit: Even though alternative or herbal remedies are not medications per se, they can still interfere with other medications and can have serious side effects if not taken correctly. Always speak with your doctor first before beginning any type of nutritional supplementation and/or herbal remedy.

Probiotics

Research into the effect of probiotics on GERD is ongoing, and much of it is positive. Studies suggest that probiotics, which contain beneficial microbes or bacteria, may help treat some digestive disorders such as GERD. What are probiotics? Probiotics are a functional component of foods that may help to boost immunity and improve overall health, especially GI health. There is promising evidence that probiotics may help treat diarrhea, prevent and treat yeast infections and urinary tract infections, treat irritable bowel syndrome, prevent and treat eczema in children, and even reduce the severity of colds and flu. Probiotics are a natural and non-digestive food ingredient that has been linked with promoting the growth of "healthy" or "friendly" bacteria in the digestive tract, just like the ones naturally found in your gut. When your body experiences low levels of these much-needed "healthy" bacteria, it can mean an overgrowth of the not-so-friendly bacteria, which can affect your health, including your digestive system. This imbalance of "good" and "bad" bacteria in turn can possibly increase your symptoms of acid reflux and GERD. Another theory currently being researched about how probiotics help GERD says that they may strengthen the lining of the gastrointestinal tract by protecting it from harmful bacteria such as H. pylori. Probiotics are also believed to help with chronic constipation, which can aggravate the symptoms of GERD, and may aide in reducing inflammation of the GI tract.

How do you boost probiotics in your diet? One way you can boost these healthy bacteria in your body is by taking probiotic supplements, which contain live microbials. Don't worry, they are friendly! These supplements come in a variety of forms, such as capsules, powders, and liquids, with the strains *bifidobacteria bifidum* and *lactobacillus acidophilus* being the most common for support of intestinal health. When choosing a probiotic supplement, always check the "best by" date, as these supplements tend to lose their potency quickly. If a product does not list a "best by" date it probably contains minimal or no live bacteria by the time of purchase and/or consumption, and therefore will not be as effective. They are usually sensitive to heat, moisture, and air, and many need to be refrigerated. Each specific probiotic appears to be effective for certain illnesses, so choosing which is best for you is important to its effectiveness. Determining how much and how often to take these supplements will depend on your doctor's recommendation, but, generally, choosing a probiotic supplement that includes 1 to 10 billion CFUs (colony forming units) once per day is suggested.

Probiotics are also plentiful in fermented dairy foods such as yogurt, which many of us already eat. These supplements and foods that contain probiotics all contain one or more of dozens of different types of probiotic organisms, with each believed to have its own benefits. If using yogurt to supplement probiotics in your diet, be sure to read the label and look for "live active cultures" or "lactobacillus acidophilus," and choose low-fat or nonfat varieties for a healthier diet.

Though research is ongoing with regard to probiotics and GERD, and it is uncertain whether they are a "cure all" for your GERD symptoms, they may be a good addition to your treatment plan. Restoring a healthy balance of intestinal bacteria can be an important aspect of your treatment for GERD. But just as with all supplements and/ or natural remedies, consult with your doctor first about your specific medical condition.

Your Nutrition Solution Tidbit: If you have heard of probiotics, chances are you have also heard of *pre*biotics. Prebiotics are non-digestible carbohydrates that act as food for probiotics. Many foods contain both prebiotics and probiotics, such as yogurt, which contains both live "good" bacteria and the fuel they need to thrive.

Calcium

Calcium is sometimes used as a natural remedy for heartburn—and it just so happens to be the active ingredient in most over-the-counter antacids. However, taking calcium in a powder form is not as much for the antacid effect as it is for tightening the LES valve, which can reduce heartburn. The best and most effective type of calcium to take is calcium citrate because of its solubility. A suggested dose is 250 milligrams, dissolved in water, after every meal and at bedtime for a total dose of 1,000 milligrams per day. Taking a calcium pill will not have the same effect and will not prevent reflux because the calcium is not instantly dissolved. Keep in mind that even though calcium is a mineral our body needs, you should not consume more than the recommended daily allowance for your age and gender. Too much calcium, especially if you are taking a calcium supplement in addition, can have other consequences. Always talk to your doctor before adding a calcium supplement to your current diet.

Magnesium

Magnesium is another mineral that may come into play in the treatment of acid reflux. Magnesium helps the sphincter or the valve at the bottom of the stomach to relax, allowing digested food to pass through and move on its way. Not getting enough magnesium can cause those gastric juices to reflux if they cannot easily pass through. The problem is that many of us don't get enough magnesium in our diets through food, and then long-term use (meaning more than a year) of prescription PPIs can cause even lower magnesium levels. If you are on any type of diuretic or beta-blocker medications for other health issues in addition to prescription PPIs, you can be at an even higher risk for magnesium deficiency. Low magnesium levels can cause unpleasant symptoms, with worsening of acid reflux being only one. Some people have found relief with a dose of about 250 mg of magnesium citrate or chelated magnesium glycinate (both highly absorbable forms) twice a day in addition to calcium citrate. Magnesium citrate can have a mild laxative effect and although chelated magnesium glycinate is less likely to cause a laxative effect, it can be more expensive. However, be sure to check with your doctor and have your levels tested before considering a magnesium supplement. Remember, not all people have the same cause for their acid reflux, and taking calcium and magnesium may only work for those whose acid reflux is related directly to the functioning of their LES. Talk to your doctor first about whether a magnesium supplement is needed and what dosage is best for you.

Your Nutrition Solution Tidbit: A few good food sources of magnesium include wheat bran, wheat germ, whole grains, almonds, pecans, walnuts, cashews, soy beans, dried pumpkin seeds, brown rice, avocado, beans, barley, green leafy vegetables, oatmeal, salmon, yogurt, potatoes, peanut butter, flaxseed, and soy milk. You need plenty in your diet, as only about 30 to 40 percent of what you consume through foods is actually absorbed into the body.

Zinc Carnosine

Zinc carnosine is an amino acid chelate (meaning it is a compound) made of zinc, an essential trace mineral; and L-carnosine, a type of amino acid found naturally in our bodies. It appears that the combination chelate is three times more effective than each ingredient individually. Zinc carnosine is a supplement that was developed and used mostly to help treat gastric ulcers. This compound appears to adhere to ulcer sites and reduce the inflammatory response to H. pylori, a bacteria found in the stomach that weakens the gastric lining and makes the stomach more susceptible to damage from gastric acid. In addition, it seems that zinc carnosine has antioxidant properties and can protect gastric mucosa from the damage of free radicals that can cause chronic diseases. Newer studies now support this supplement's beneficial effects on acid reflux by helping to inhibit gastric acid secretion. The common dosage for zinc carnosine is 75 milligrams per day between meals, but check with your doctor first.

Your Nutrition Solution Tidbit: The best food sources for the trace mineral zinc are oysters, meat, crab, eggs, other seafood, black-eyed peas, and some beans.

Digestive Enzymes

Digestive enzymes occur naturally in our bodies and are meant to aide, along with stomach acid, in the digestion and breakdown of food into smaller, more absorbable components. Enzymes called "amylase" break down starches into sugar molecules; "protease" enzymes break down proteins into amino acids, and "lipase" enzymes break down fat into its absorbable form. Digestive enzymes go hand-in-hand with gastric acids because it is the acids that activate the all-important enzymes. Enzymes can be found not only in our bodies but also in some fresh foods; cooked and processed foods don't have enough enzymes and therefore require more from your body. If your body comes up short on enzymes this can delay gastric emptying, which in turn can play a role in worsening acid reflux symptoms. There is no concrete scientific evidence that digestive enzymes are useful for GERD, but for some people they have shown promising results in alleviating symptoms and improving overall digestive health. A vast variety of digestive enzyme products are on the market today. Look for enzyme products that contain all of the necessary enzymes for breaking down all of the food components, including lipase (for fat), protease (for protein), and amylase (for carbohydrates). Taking digestive enzymes before meals or at least within about 30 minutes of consuming a meal will be most beneficial.

Your Nutrition Solution Tidbit: The food chemical codex (FCC) is a compendium of standards used internationally for the quality and purity of food ingredients such as preservatives, flavorings, colorings, and nutrients. The United States Pharmacopoeia (USP) publishes the FCC and also conducts verification programs for dietary supplement products and ingredients. The FCC is the accepted standard of the U.S. Food and Drug Administration (FDA). If a product meets all of the requirements of the USP it can display the USP Verified Dietary Supplement Mark on their labels. The system that is used to determine enzyme potency by the American food industry is derived from the FCC. FCC units measure the amount of substrate that is digested in a certain amount of time by a specific enzyme. For example, if the enzyme lipase has a USP of 1,000 units per milligram (mg), that would mean that for every mg of lipase that you consume it will digest 1,000 USP units of fat in a specific amount of time.

Betaine HCL

As discussed in Chapter 1, low stomach acid can be a culprit of acid reflux and GERD. If it seems you have tried everything and your reflux is not responding, you should speak with your doctor about possible testing and diagnosis for this problem. It is much more common than you may think. There are several tests your doctor can use in the office to test the level of your stomach acid, and there are a few at-home tests you can experiment with as well. (Check out Chapter 7 for these at-home tests.) If you are found to have low stomach acid the treatment will most likely be to replace that lowered stomach acid with a supplement until the root cause is found. The most common treatment for low stomach acid is a supplement called Betaine HCL (hydrochloride). This supplement helps to increase the level of hydrochloric acid in the stomach that is essential for the proper digestion and absorption of nutrients from the foods we consume. We need normal levels of hydrochloric acid in our stomachs to completely digest proteins and absorb amino acids, the building blocks of protein. We also need this acid to extract vitamin B12 from the foods we eat. Betaine HCL helps to restore proper acid levels in the stomach, which are required for maintaining healthy GI function. Betaine HCL is typically taken in a pill form at doses typically ranging from 325 to 640 milligrams at each meal. It may be helpful to choose a supplement that also contains enzymes such as pancreatic enzymes or pepsin. Ask your doctor which supplement is best for you, and at what dosage. If you are taking any type of anti-inflammatory medicines ask your doctor before taking a Betaine HCL supplement.

Glutamine

Glutamine is an amino acid (one of the building blocks of protein) that naturally occurs in the body and can be found in some food sources. It is in fact the most abundant amino acid in your body. Glutamine acts as an anti-inflammatory that can help reduce intestinal inflammation that is commonly associated with acid reflux. Glutamine helps to protect your gastrointestinal tract lining, which is known as the mucosa. Its protective and healing properties may benefit the lower esophagus, stomach, and upper small intestine—all of the parts of the GI system that are vulnerable to erosive damage in people who experience GERD. Once triggers of GERD are pinpointed and addressed, glutamine can begin to help the healing of the lining of the gut.

The common form of this amino acid in dietary supplements is L-glutamine. Doses of 500 milligrams, one to three times daily, are generally considered safe. Higher doses of L-glutamine are also thought to be safe and may be prescribed by a healthcare provider if needed. You can find L-glutamine in powder, capsule, tablet, or liquid forms. If using the powdered form, do not add to hot beverages as the heat will destroy the amino acid. If you have liver or kidney disease or Reye syndrome you should avoid glutamine so check with your doctor first and inquire about the best dosage to take for use with GERD. In addition, L-glutamine can interact with some medications, so, again, check with your doctor before taking.

Your Nutrition Solution Tidbit: Glutamine can also be found in some dietary sources, such as animal and plant proteins including beef, pork, poultry, milk, yogurt, cottage cheese, raw spinach, and cabbage.

Slippery Elm Bark

Slippery elm bark (also known as Ulmus rubra) is an herb that has been used for centuries but has recently been touted as a natural way to treat acid reflux by protecting the gastrointestinal tract against ulcers and excess acidity. It may also help to reduce inflammation in the mouth, throat, stomach, and intestines. Slippery elm contains mucilage, a substance that forms a protective coating over the irritated or inflamed mucosa. In addition, this herb contains a high amount of antioxidants, which may also offer some protection to the digestive tract. To make this supplement, the inner bark of the slippery elm tree is dried and powdered. It can be found in tablets or capsules, lozenges, and also as a fine powder for making teas or extracts. Recommended doses, for adults only, includes: for tea, pouring 2 cups boiling water over 4 grams (about 2 tablespoons) of finely powdered bark and steeping for about five minutes, consumed three times per day; for capsules, taking 400 to 500 milligrams, three to four times daily for four to eight weeks with a full glass of water is recommended. Because slippery elm coats the digestive tract, it may have a tendency to slow down the absorption of other medications and/or herbs. It is best to take this herb at least two hours before or after taking other herbs and/or medications. Always ask your doctor before taking any herbal supplement, and ask what dosage is safest for you. Ask your doctor about safety if you are pregnant or breastfeeding.

Your Nutrition Solution Tidbit: Keep in mind that even though herbs are "natural," they can still trigger side effects and can interact with other herbs, supplements, and/or medications. For these reasons, you should use caution and speak with your doctor before taking any type of herbal supplement.

Deglycyrrhizinated Licorice (DGL)

DGL is an herbal licorice extract, not to be confused with licorice candy! It is known that the glycyrrhizin in licorice root can cause issues with high blood pressure and fluid retention, and create possible problems for those who have diabetes. So long-term use of the licorice root is definitely a concern. However, in the deglycyrrhizinated form, substantial parts of the glycyrrhizin have been removed, making it a safer option for more people and for a longer period of time if needed.

DGL is frequently used to treat indigestion and heartburn as well as ulcer and esophagitis symptoms by increasing the mucous coating in the stomach, lower esophagus, and intestinal tract, which in turn protects these tissues from irritation caused by gastric acids. Slowly chewing two DGL tablets, about 400 milligrams per tablet, before or between meals and at bedtime, may help relieve symptoms of acid reflux and can also aide by boosting enzyme production, allowing for quicker and better digestion. DGL can be found in a powdered form, which should also be taken between meals. Talk to your doctor before taking DGL to discuss proper dosage and possible side effects.

chapter 3

your 5-step nutrition
and lifestyle solution

What we put into our bodies nutritionally and how we treat our bodies physically can have a huge impact on our overall health—and that includes acid reflux and GERD. This Chapter will detail five steps you can follow to get to the root of your acid reflux problems and start feeling better. Treatment for acid reflux and GERD is quite individualized, so it is important to do what works for *you*! The key is to be hands-on and to make changes that will remedy your problem for the long term. You may read some of these solutions and think, *I already know that.* But *knowing* and *doing* are two completely different things! All five of these steps tackle things you *do* have control over. Now is the time to empower yourself to take action!

Step 1: Modify Your Eating and Lifestyle Behaviors

Following are some eating and lifestyle behavior tips that can start to control your acid reflux symptoms immediately. It is up to you to implement these positive changes in your everyday life.

- Raise the head of your bed 6 to 8 inches by placing blocks of wood or bricks under the bedposts. Using extra pillows is not effective in helping to reduce acid reflux; it will only raise your head and give you a neck ache. If lifting the bed is not possible try a foam wedge that will elevate your entire upper body and not just your head.

- Reach and maintain a healthy weight (you will find more information on this later in this chapter).

- Avoid alcoholic beverages.

- If you smoke, stop smoking! There are endless reasons why you should quit smoking, but as far as GERD goes, nicotine relaxes the LES, allowing gastric acids to reflux back into the esophagus and cause heartburn. Furthermore, cigarettes promote additional acid production in the stomach.

- Forget the rule of three meals a day and eat smaller meals more often throughout the day. Eating too much at one sitting can overwhelm the LES, causing reflux. If you need help doing this, try using a smaller plate as a way to ensure you eat smaller portions and don't go back for seconds. If you are at a healthy weight then you can eat the same number of calories throughout the day but spread them out so you don't eat too much at any one sitting. If you are overweight and looking to lose weight this can have a dual effect. Eat smaller meals to lower your calorie intake.

- Slow down, stop eating on the run, and eat at a slower pace. Chew your food thoroughly, and don't rush. Try putting your fork down between bites. Too much food in the stomach in a short period of time can lead to reflux. Those smaller portions you are now eating will go a lot further if you slow down.

- Eat a dry starch at night such as a small baked potato, crackers, or dry whole-wheat toast with NO liquids an hour before bedtime. The dry starch, with no liquid, may help to absorb the gastric juices and keep it from refluxing back up into the reclining esophagus. Carbohydrates before bedtime feeds seratonin, which turns into melatonin and makes for a good night's sleep too.

- Time your meals around your exercise routine so that you wait at least two hours after a meal to exercise or engage in other intense physical activity. Working out too soon after eating can trigger heartburn.

- Drink beverages between meals instead of with meals so you don't bloat your stomach and cause possible reflux.

- Drink more water, not during meals, but between meals. Opt for water in place of caffeine and/or sugar-containing beverages and carbonated drinks. Carbonated beverages tend to bloat your stomach, forcing acid to back up your esophagus. Getting rid of the calorie-laden drinks will help with weight loss as well.

- Refrain from wearing tight-fitting clothing and belts. Wearing something that is looser-fitting and comfortable will ensure you are not putting extra pressure on your abdomen, which can contribute to reflux symptoms.

- Avoid lying down, bending over, or straining right after eating. Do not lie down for at least three hours after eating a meal. You will need to be mindful of what time you eat before going to bed.

- Simply improving your posture can help food and gastric acids stay in the stomach where they belong instead of spilling into the esophagus. (And who couldn't use a reminder to stand up straighter?)

- Attempt to lie on your left side while sleeping. Research has shown that sleeping on your stomach can worsen symptoms of acid reflux. And sleeping on your left side seems to be more helpful then sleeping on your right. It is easy and worth a try!

- Evaluate, along with your doctor, other medications you may be taking. Some common medications can make GERD worse, such as aspirin and other NSAID painkillers and medications for high blood pressure. Talk to your doctor and pharmacist about the medications you are taking and if any of them worsen or cause symptoms of acid reflux. Ask about possible alternatives that won't.

Step 2: Eat a Healthier Diet

I am sure this one doesn't come as a surprise. But instead of simply thinking about changing your diet, it is time to seriously review your current eating habits, become more educated, and make some positive changes. Consuming an overall healthier diet is not only going to help you to control your acid reflux symptoms and possibly get to the root of your problem, but it is going to improve your health and your weight as well—a giant plus when trying to manage acid reflux and GERD! The good news is that you have a wealth of nutrition information on how to eat and live healthier right at your fingertips with the USDA's Website ChooseMyPlate.gov and the Dietary Guidelines for Americans (*www.health.gov/dietaryguidelines*). Reading them is the perfect first step to help you make healthier nutritional and lifestyle choices in order to begin reducing your acid reflux symptoms.

Both ChooseMyPlate.gov and the Dietary Guidelines for Americans are issued and updated jointly by the Department of Agriculture (USDA) and the Department of Health and Human Services (HHS) every five years. The guidelines work hand-in-hand to provide the most current science-based advice for all Americans 2 years of age and older. They are available for all Americans so that we can educate ourselves as to what good nutrition is and how we can make healthier choices. The key is not to only read both of these educational components but also to implement them in your everyday life.

The Dietary Guidelines for Americans

The newest set of Dietary Guidelines for Americans focuses on three major goals that together emphasize a total lifestyle approach:

1. Balance calories with physical activity to manage weight.

2. Consume more healthy foods and nutrients such as fruits, vegetables, whole grains, fat-free and low-fat dairy products, and seafood.

3. Consume fewer foods with sodium (salt), saturated fats, trans fats, cholesterol, added sugars, and refined grains.

These guidelines are intended to aide Americans in maintaining a healthy weight, reducing the risk of chronic disease, and promoting good overall health. The current Dietary Guidelines for Americans include 23 key recommendations for the general population and six additional key recommendations for specific groups whose needs may differ slightly, such as pregnant women. These recommendations are meant to help you reach the three major goals set by the guidelines. I will summarize the 23 general recommendations here, but you are highly encouraged to visit *www.cnpp.usda.gov/Publications/DietaryGuidelines/2010/ PolicyDoc/PolicyDoc.pdf* to read the 2010 guidelines in full detail.

These recommendations are key to adopting healthier lifestyle habits that will help to reduce your symptoms of acid reflux, reduce your risk for numerous chronic diseases, and increase your chances for a longer, healthier life. It is all up to *you!*

Balancing Calories to Manage Weight

1. **Prevent and/or reduce overweight and obesity through improved eating and physical activity behaviors.** These are lifestyle changes you have control of that will not only help you to manage your weight and your health but your acid reflux issues as well.

2. **Control total calorie intake to manage body weight. For people who are overweight or obese, this will mean consuming fewer calories from foods and beverages.** Balancing your calorie intake over time is the key to weight management and keeping weight off. This means balancing the calories you burn through physical activity with the number of calories you consume. If these numbers equal, you will maintain your weight; if they shift to the negative, you will lose weight; if they shift to the positive, you will begin to gain weight. So the goal here is to get control over this balance of calories in and calories out, and shift it in your favor.

3. **Increase physical activity and reduce time spent in sedentary behaviors.** Physical activity has all types of health and even mental benefits, and it is essential in the calorie-balance equation for weight management. In spite of that, less then 5 percent of American adults participate in at least 30 minutes of physical activity each day, and only a few more meet the recommended weekly goal of at least 150 minutes. We will discuss exercise more a bit later in this chapter.

4. **Maintain appropriate calorie balance during each stage of life—childhood, adolescence, adulthood, pregnancy and breastfeeding, and older age.** Maintaining the calorie-in and calorie-out equation will not be a temporary situation to lose weight. It will be a lifelong adjustment to maintain your healthy weight. It is much easier to balance this equation and maintain your healthy weight than to gain unwanted weight and then have to lose it. Lifestyle and eating habits need to change permanently in order to maintain a healthy weight and improved health.

Foods and Food Components to Reduce

5. **Reduce daily sodium intake to less than 2,300 milligrams (mg).** For persons who are 51 and older, African American, or who have hypertension, diabetes, or chronic kidney disorder, reduce intake to 1,500 mg. The 1,500 mg recommendation applies to about half of the U.S. population,

including children and the majority of adults.
Most Americans consume far more sodium than
what is recommended and what our bodies need. In
fact, on average, Americans consume around 3,400
milligrams per day. Research has indicated that as
sodium levels decrease so do blood pressure rates.
When our blood pressure is in the normal range
we decrease our risk for cardiovascular disease,
kidney disease, and congestive heart failure. Most
of the sodium we ingest is consumed as salt (sodium chloride) added to foods for various reasons.
You can help decrease your sodium intake by:

⊠ Reading the Nutrition Facts label (or food label) for information on the sodium content
of foods you purchase and choosing ones that
are lower in sodium. The Percent Daily Value
will tell you how much of your daily allowance
for sodium the food takes up in one serving.
So if a food states 50% Daily Value, you are
going to consume half of your sodium allowance for the entire day.

⊠ Consuming more fresh foods and fewer processed foods, which are usually quite high
in sodium. Fresh foods are naturally low in
sodium.

⊠ Eating more home-prepared foods, for which
you control the amount of sodium used. Use
little to no salt or salt-containing seasonings.
Instead use spices and herbs when cooking or
eating foods at home.

⌐ When eating out, asking that salt not be added to your food or ordering lower-sodium options if they are available.

⌐ Taking the salt shaker off the dinner table!

6. **Consume less than 10 percent of calories from saturated fatty acids by replacing them with monounsaturated and polyunsaturated fatty acids.** Added fats can add loads of unnecessary calories to foods. Choosing the wrong types of fat too often can cause a host of health problems such as heart disease, stroke, and high cholesterol. Fats are categorized as *saturated* or unhealthy fats and *monounsaturated and polyunsaturated* or healthy fats. The type of fats you consume influences health risks more than the total amount of fat you consume, so it is important to choose fat-containing foods wisely. Saturated fats come from animal foods and products cooked or baked with animal fats such as baked goods, beef, chicken, pork, and dairy products. Monounsaturated fats are considered a healthy fat and can be found in plant foods such as canola, safflower, and olive oils as well as avocado, olives, peanuts, pecans, sesame seeds, and peanut butter. Polyunsaturated fats can be found in plant foods such as corn, soybean, and cottonseed oils as well as walnuts, pumpkin seeds, and sunflower seeds.

You can help decrease unhealthy fats by:

⌐ Making major sources of saturated fats such as cakes, cookies, ice cream, pizza, cheese, sausage, burgers, and hot dogs occasional choices and not everyday foods.

➢ Selecting lean cuts of meat and poultry and choosing fat-free or low-fat milk, yogurt, and cheeses.

➢ Switching from solid fats to liquid oils when preparing foods at home.

➢ Reading food labels before purchasing foods and choosing ones with lower saturated fat contents.

7. **Consume less than 300 mg per day of dietary cholesterol.** We need cholesterol in our bodies for a few essential functions, but our body makes more than enough for these specific purposes. Therefore we need very little in the way of cholesterol-containing foods in our daily diet. Major sources of cholesterol in the American diet include whole eggs, chicken, beef, pork, and burgers as well as reduced-fat or whole-fat dairy products, fast foods, and snack products such as chips and baked goods. Too much dietary cholesterol in our diet can lead to high levels of LDL or the "bad" cholesterol, which in turn can lead to cardiovascular disease and stroke.

You can help decrease dietary cholesterol by:

➢ Filling your daily diet with fruits, vegetables, lean meats, fish, fat-free dairy foods, and whole grains.

➢ Switching out solid or saturated fats such as butter with healthier fats such as olive oil.

➢ Looking for products that are specifically made for low-cholesterol diets.

ℵ Substituting some of your whole eggs with egg whites (which contain no cholesterol) or egg substitutes.

ℵ Checking food labels and choosing foods with lower cholesterol contents.

8. **Keep trans fatty acid consumption as low as possible, especially by limiting foods that contain synthetic sources of trans fats, such as partially hydrogenated oils, and by limiting other solid fats.** Trans fats are unsaturated fats that differ in their structure from other unsaturated fats and therefore are not considered healthy. Trans fats are not essential in our diets. They can be found naturally in some foods and are formed during processing (hydrogenation) in others. It is the trans fats that are formed during processing that tend to be the most damaging to our health. To find trans fats in foods check the food label and/or look for the words "hydrogenated oil" or "partially hydrogenated oil" in the ingredient list.

9. **Reduce the intake of calories from solid fats and added sugars.** Research tells us that the intake of saturated fats and trans fats can increase our risk for chronic disease, especially cardiovascular disease. Most fats with a high percentage of saturated and trans fats are solid at room temperature, and therefore are referred to as "solid fats."

Sugar can be found naturally in some foods, including *lactose* in most dairy products and *fructose* in fruits. However, the majority of sugars found in the average American diet are added sugars.

These sugars are added in processing, preparation, or at the table to sweeten and improve palatability. They are also added as a preservative and to provide texture, body, viscosity, and browning capacity to foods. Although our body cannot determine the difference between natural and added sugars, the key is that foods with natural sugars usually contain the whole package of nutrients and other healthful components such as fiber. On the other hand, most foods with added sugars often supply calories with little to no essential nutrients, and no fiber. You may see added sugars on food labels termed *high fructose corn syrup, white sugar, brown sugar, corn syrup, raw sugar, malt syrup, fructose sweetener, liquid fructose, honey, molasses,* and *crystal dextrose.* The major sources of added sugars in the American diet include soft drinks, energy drinks, sports drinks, baked goods, sugar-sweetened drinks, dairy-based drinks, and of course candy. Reducing the consumption of added sugars can lower the calorie content of the diet without the worry of leaving out essential nutrients.

Solid fats and added sugars are a particular concern in the American diet because both have been found to be consumed in excessive amounts. Their intake should be limited. Together, these two food components contribute a substantial amount of calories to our diets—35 percent of total daily calories—without contributing to our nutritional needs. This makes them very dangerous when it comes to managing weight. When consumed in excess, foods that contain solid fats and added sugars begin to take the place of foods with essential vitamins, minerals, and fiber. Reducing the consumption of these foods allows us to increase our intake of nutrient-dense foods without going over our total daily calorie needs.

You can help decrease solid fats and added sugars by:

- ✄ Focusing on eating the most nutrient-dense (or nutrition-filled) forms of foods from all of the food groups.

- ✄ Limiting solid fats and added sugars when cooking or eating by trimming fat from meat, using less butter or stick margarine in favor of healthy oils, and using less table sugar.

- ✄ Choosing smaller portions if consuming foods with solid fats and/or added sugars such as baked goods, soft drinks, and other sugar-sweetened beverages.

- ✄ Drinking water instead of sugary drinks.

10. **Limit the consumption of foods that contain refined grains, especially refined grain foods that contain solid fats, added sugars, and sodium.** We have heard time and time again that whole grains are better for us than refined grains, but what exactly is the difference? Basically, grains start off as whole and are then processed or refined. During this process, the grain is stripped of many vitamins, minerals, and fiber. To rectify this problem most refined grains are then enriched with iron, thiamin (vitamin B1), riboflavin (vitamin B2), niacin, and

folic acid before being used as an ingredient in other foods. This returns some, but not all of the nutrients that were removed during the refining process. Dietary fiber and some vitamins and minerals that are there to begin with in the whole grain are never able to be added back to the refined grain. Enriched refined grains products do provide some vitamins and minerals, but when they are consumed beyond recommended levels, they provide excess calories with not enough nutritional intake. In addition, many refined food products contain solid fats and added sugars, such as cookies and cakes. Refined grains include white breads, tortillas, pizza crust, white rice, pasta, and baked goods such as cookies, cakes, donuts, and other desserts. Whole grains include whole-wheat or whole-grain breads, brown rice, wild rice, whole-wheat pasta, and whole-grain cereals. The goal should be to eat at least half of your grains as whole grains and to limit refined grains that contain solids fats and added sugars as much as possible.

11. **If alcohol is consumed, it should be consumed in moderation—up to one drink per day for women and two drinks per day for men—and only by adults of legal drinking age.** Approximately 50 percent of American adults are regular drinkers, with 29 percent reporting that they occasionally binge drink. The consumption of alcohol can have beneficial effects or detrimental effects depending on how much is consumed and how often, as well as one's age and health issues. Alcohol consumption

may have beneficial effects when consumed in moderation, especially red wine. However, it is never recommended to start drinking if you are a non-drinker. Heavy drinking, on the other hand, has absolutely no health benefits, and can cause a wealth of health issues including cirrhosis of the liver, high blood pressure, stroke, type 2 diabetes, and cancer of the upper gastrointestinal tract and colon. In time heavy drinking can also lead to an increase in body weight and can impair both short- and long-term cognitive function. It is also important to mention here that any amount of alcohol can be a trigger for acid reflux for many people.

Your Nutrition Solution Tidbit: *Moderate alcohol consumption* is defined as up to one drink per day for women and up to two drinks per day for men. *Heavy or excessive alcohol consumption* is defined as more than three drinks on any day or more than seven per week for women, and more than four drinks on any day or more than 14 per week for men. *Alcohol binge drinking* is defined as four or more drinks for women and five or more drinks for men in a two-hour period.

Foods and Nutrients to Increase

12. **Increase vegetable and fruit intake.** Eating more fruits and vegetables is necessary for a few reasons: First, they are packed with tons of essential

nutrients, many of which are under-consumed by most Americans. Second, research shows that eating fruits and vegetables is associated with the reduced risk of many chronic diseases. Eating at least 2 1/2 cups of fruits and vegetables daily is associated with a reduced risk of cardiovascular disease such as heart attack and stroke. Fruits and vegetables may even help to protect against certain types of cancer. Third, there is the added benefit of most fruits and veggies being relatively low in calories. If you swap out higher-calorie snacks with fruits and vegetables you are bound to lose a few pounds.

13. **Eat a variety of vegetables, especially dark green, red, and orange vegetables, and beans and peas.** Mom always told you to eat your spinach, but little did she know how beneficial it really is. The more color, the more nutritional value! And don't forget about the beans and peas. Beans and peas, or legumes, are excellent sources of protein, iron, zinc, potassium, folate, and dietary fiber, and are low in fat and calories. They are such a great source of protein and nutrients that they can be considered as both a vegetable and a protein food. Consider swapping out meat a few times a week for a main dish focused on beans.

14. **Consume at least half of all grains as whole grains. Increase whole-grain intake by replacing refined grains with whole grains.** I discussed this in detail earlier. It doesn't take much to include more whole grains in your daily diet. If you get at

least half of your grains from whole grains you are making a positive and beneficial change. Switch your breads to whole-wheat or whole-grain varieties, choose cereal for breakfast that is labeled whole-grain, and swap out white rice for brown rice. These are simple changes that can make a big difference.

Your Nutrition Solution Tidbit: Whole grains are consumed as either a single food such as brown rice or popcorn or as an ingredient in a food such as buckwheat or bulgur. Other whole grains include millet, oatmeal, quinoa, rolled oats, wild rice, whole-grain barley, whole rye, and whole wheat. It's nice to know that even popcorn is a whole grain and can be healthy if you don't top it with loads of butter and salt! When choosing whole-grain foods, look for the word *whole* on the label or in the ingredient list to ensure it is actually a whole grain. For example, bread labeled simply "Wheat Bread" is not whole-grain. These breads usually contain enriched wheat flour that does not have enough of the whole grain left in it to be labeled as a whole grain. It should state "whole-wheat or whole-grain bread" to be beneficial and count as a whole grain. Look for the whole-grain ingredient in the product to be first or second on the list.

15. **Increase intake of fat-free or low-fat milk and milk products, such as milk, yogurt, cheese, or fortified soy beverages.** Milk and milk products provide calcium, vitamin D, and potassium to our diet. This food group is essential for good bone health and is also linked to a reduced risk of cardiovascular disease and type 2 diabetes as well as lower blood pressure in adults. Recommended amounts are three cups per day.

16. **Choose a variety of protein foods, which include seafood, lean meat and poultry, eggs, beans and peas, soy products, and unsalted nuts and seeds.** In addition to providing protein, these foods also supply plenty of B vitamins including niacin, thiamin, riboflavin, and B6, as well as vitamin E, iron, zinc, and magnesium to our daily diets. The key is to consume a variety of these foods for your best nutritional intake.

17. **Increase the amount and variety of seafood consumed by choosing seafood in place of some meat and poultry.** Seafood includes fish such as salmon, tuna, trout, and tilapia, and shellfish such as shrimp, lobster, crab, and oysters. Seafood is a much healthier option as a protein source due to the type of fat it contains, which is the "good" or healthy fat. Fish and shellfish contribute many nutrients, but most important are the omega-3 fatty acids eicosapentaenoic acid (EPA) and docosahexaenoic acid (DHA). Research shows that

consuming about 8 ounces of seafood per week will provide enough EPA and DHA to help lower the risk of cardiovascular disease.

Your Nutrition Solution Tidbit: Because seafood contains varying levels of mercury (some more than others), the FDA and EPA (Environmental Protection Agency) have issued a fish-consumption advisory for women who may become pregnant, pregnant women, nursing mothers, and young children as follows:

By following these three recommendations for selecting and eating fish or shellfish, women and young children will receive the benefits of eating fish and shellfish and be confident that they have reduced their exposure to the harmful effects of mercury.

Do not eat Shark, Swordfish, King Mackerel, or Tilefish because they contain high levels of mercury.

Eat up to 12 ounces (two average meals) a week of a variety of fish and shellfish that are lower in mercury.

Five of the most commonly eaten fish that are low in mercury are shrimp, canned light tuna, salmon, pollock, and catfish.

Another commonly eaten fish, albacore ("white") tuna has more mercury than canned light tuna. So, when choosing your two meals of fish and shellfish, you may eat up to 6 ounces (one average meal) of albacore tuna per week.

Check local advisories about the safety of fish caught by family and friends in your local lakes, rivers, and coastal areas. If no advice is available, eat up to 6 ounces (one average meal) per week of fish you catch from local waters, but don't consume any other fish during that week.

Source: www.epa.gov/hg/advisories.htm

18. **Replace protein foods that are higher in solid fats with choices that are lower in solid fats and calories and/or are sources of oils.** The fats found in meat, poultry, and eggs are considered solid fats (or the "bad" fats) whereas the fats in seafood, nuts, and seeds are considered oils (or the "good" fats). The key is to choose lean forms of meats and poultry to decrease solid fats and to increase your consumption of seafood, beans, soy products, nuts, and seeds as a protein source.

19. **Use oils to replace solid fats where possible.** Fats are not considered a food group but they are emphasized in the Dietary Guidelines because they supply essential fatty acids and vitamin E to our diets. Replacing some of the saturated fats with unsaturated fats can help to lower both total cholesterol and low-density lipoprotein (LDL, the "bad" cholesterol). Unsaturated fats such as oils can be found naturally in some foods such as olives, nuts, avocados, and seafood. Some oils are extracted

from plants, such as canola, olive, corn, safflower, soybean, and sunflower oils. You can also find oils in oil-based salad dressings, soft margarines with no trans fatty acids, and mayonnaise. The key is to get more oils and less solid fats and to also keep in mind that whether fats are healthy or unhealthy they are all a concentrated source of calories, so use them all in moderation.

20. **Choose foods that provide more potassium, dietary fiber, calcium, and vitamin D, which are nutrients of concern in American diets. These foods include vegetables, fruits, whole grains, and milk and milk products.** All of these nutrients are emphasized in the Dietary Guidelines because on average most Americans do not consume enough of them.

Dietary potassium can help to lower blood pressure for those with hypertension, reduce the risk of developing kidney stones, and decrease bone loss. Potassium can be found in just about all the food groups but especially in fruits, vegetables, and dairy products.

Dietary fiber is a non-digestible form of carbohydrates. Consuming enough fiber may help to reduce the risk of cardiovascular disease, obesity, and type 2 diabetes. Children and adults should get enough fiber in order to promote healthy lipid profiles (such as cholesterol and triglyceride levels) and glucose (blood sugar) tolerance, and ensure normal gastrointestinal function. Women should get somewhere around 25 grams per day and men should get 38 grams per day for optimal health. Most Americans don't even come close. Fiber naturally occurs in plant sources such as beans and peas, vegetables, fruits, whole grains, bran, and nuts. Use the Nutrition Facts label on foods to determine fiber content and choose foods that provide more fiber.

Calcium is needed for optimal bone health. Calcium also serves a vital role in nerve transmission, constriction and dilation of blood vessels, and muscle contraction. Many Americans have low bone density due to low calcium intake, which puts them at higher risk for osteoporosis (a brittle bone disease that occurs later in life especially in women) and bone fractures. Fat-free or low-fat milk and milk products are the best sources of calcium. Some plant foods such as almonds and dark green leafy vegetables can also contribute calcium, but consuming enough of these plant foods to meet recommendations would be tough. It is vital for those who do not consume dairy products to carefully replace them with other food sources of calcium, including fortified foods, and possibly supplements, but speak with your doctor first.

Vitamin D status is important for good health. Adequate amounts of vitamin D are needed to help reduce the risk of bone fractures. Not only can we get vitamin D from some of the fortified foods we eat, such as milk and milk products, some yogurts, breakfast cereals, margarine, and orange juice, but we are also able to obtain vitamin D from sunlight on the skin, which enables the body to make vitamin D.

Building Healthy Eating Patterns

21. **Select an eating pattern that meets nutrient needs over time at an appropriate calorie level.** There are plenty of healthy eating patterns out there that apply most of the recommendations from the Dietary Guidelines. The USDA Food Patterns along with the DASH Eating Plan (Dietary Approaches to Stop Hypertension) and the Mediterranean Diet are just a few. Individuals are able to adopt these healthy eating plans to suit their personal and cultural preferences.

22. **Account for all foods and beverages consumed and assess how they fit within a total healthy eating pattern.** Just about all foods and beverages can somehow fit into a healthy eating pattern. The key is to first add all of the food and nutrients you need and then to fit in some of the others where possible.

23. **Follow food safety recommendations when preparing and eating foods to reduce the risk of food-borne illnesses.** Always follow safety recommendations when preparing storing foods. Foodborne illness affects more than a whopping 76 million individuals in the United States yearly, which leads to 325,000 hospitalizations and 5,000 deaths. Keep

you and your family safe by cleaning your hands and food-contact surfaces, as well as vegetables and fruits. Separate raw, cooked, and ready-to-eat foods while shopping, storing, and preparing foods. Be sure to cook foods to a safe temperature and refrigerate perishable foods promptly. Prevent cross-contamination by using different cutting boards, utensils, and dishes for raw and cooked meats. In addition, avoid foods that pose a high risk of food-borne illness such as unpasteurized milk, cheeses, and juices; raw or undercooked animal foods such as seafood, beef, poultry, pork, and eggs, as well as raw sprouts.

Source: USDA Center for Nutrition Policy and Promotion, Dietary Guidelines for Americans, www. cnpp.usda.gov/DGAs2010-PolicyDocument.htm

ChooseMyPlate.gov

ChooseMyPlate.gov is a fairly new Website that showcases the newer icon MyPlate, which took the place of the Food Guide Pyramid in 2010. MyPlate works hand-in-hand with the Dietary Guidelines for Americans to help people:

- Make smarter choices from each food group
- Find a healthy balance between food and physical activity
- Get the most nutrition out of calories consumed
- Stay within daily calorie needs

The MyPlate icon is a familiar mealtime visual that emphasizes the five food groups, which are the foundation of a healthy diet. It divides the dinner plate into four sections, for fruits, vegetables, grains, and proteins, with a fifth, smaller plate to one side for dairy foods. MyPlate illustrates these food groups as separate colors and different sizes on the plate. For example, the fruit (red) and vegetable (green) portions make up half of the plate to emphasize the recommendation that fruits and vegetables should make up at least half of every meal.

Other key suggestions from the MyPlate guide include:

Food to Increase:

※ Make half your plate fruits and vegetables

※ Switch to fat-free or low-fat (1%) milk

※ Make at least half of your grains whole-grains

※ Go lean with protein

Foods to Reduce:

※ Compare sodium (salt) in foods like soup, bread, and frozen meals, and choose foods with lower numbers

※ Drink water instead of sugary drinks

Balancing Calories:

※ Enjoy your food, but eat less

※ Avoid oversized portions

※ Find a balance between food and physical activity

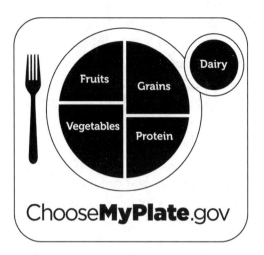

In addition to the MyPlate icon, ChooseMyPlate.gov is full of helpful tools to start you on the right path to a healthier diet.

The Website includes the following sections.

- ⋈ **MyPlate.** This section dives into each food group included in the MyPlate Icon in detail and provides you with all of the information you need to eat healthier once and for all.

- ⋈ **Weight Management & Calories.** This section is dedicated to helping you understand how calories are involved in losing weight.

- ⋈ **Physical Activity.** This section provides you with all of the important information on physical activity and how to use it to your advantage.

- ⋈ **SuperTracker & Other Tools.** The SuperTracker is a tool to help you plan, analyze, and track your diet as well as your physical activity. You can find out what and how much to eat; track the foods you consume, the physical activity you perform, and your weight; and personalize your plan with goal-setting, virtual coaching, and journaling. The **Daily Food Plans and Worksheets** is another helpful tool that provides you with food group targets including what and how much to eat within your calorie allowance. Your daily food plan is personalized and based on your age, gender, height, weight, and physical activity level. It also includes a worksheet to help you keep track. Information is also included for pregnant women and preschoolers as well. If you want something a bit more advanced you can create a personal daily food plan using the SuperTracker's MyPlan. You will need to create a profile and you are able to save it if you want. Then you can use some or all of the SuperTracker's other helpful features. Other helpful tools in this section include Calories Burn Chart, Calories Count Chart for Mixed Dishes, Empty Calories Chart, Solids Fat Chart, BMI Calculator, Portion Distortion, and Food Labeling.

This Website has all of the information you need to start eating a healthier diet. And if you think that eating a healthier diet isn't part of the solution to treating acid reflux, you would be very wrong! Try it and find out just how much it will help!

Source: USDA ChooseMyPlate.gov, www.choosemyplate.gov

Step 3: Reach a Healthy Weight

Research has proven again and again that excess body weight can lead to a host of health issues—of which acid reflux and GERD are just a few. Excess body fat can put unwanted pressure around your belly, pushing it up and causing acid to back up into your esophagus. The added pressure impacts (lower esophageal sphincter) LES that we know joins the stomach and esophagus, causing it to relax and allow the gastric juices from the stomach to flow up into the esophagus. In addition, excess body weight can impair the body's ability to empty the stomach efficiently and quickly. Similar to modifying your eating and lifestyle behaviors and choosing an overall healthier diet, reaching and maintaining a healthy weight is within your control. The bottom line is that if you are overweight or obese you can help ease your heartburn symptoms by losing some of those unwanted pounds. As a bonus you will boost your overall health! If you are already at a healthy weight then the goal is to maintain that weight. If you are overweight or obese then the goal is to slowly and steadily lose weight in a healthy manner, no more than 1 to 2 pounds per week. Always check with your doctor first to discuss the weight-loss strategy that is best for you.

Determining Your Healthy Weight

Let's say you know you need to lose weight, but you wonder, *Exactly how much? How do I know what my healthy weight really is?* BMI or Body Mass Index is one way to determine if your extra pounds translate into greater health risk. BMI is the measurement of your weight relative to your height and can determine whether you are at a healthy weight or if your weight may be contributing to poor health, including acid reflux. Keep in mind that BMI is not a measurement of body fat; therefore, it can sometimes misclassify people. For example, people with a lot of muscle mass may have a BMI that shows too high because BMI doesn't measure exact body fat and doesn't take into consideration that the majority of their body weight is coming from muscle. It can do the opposite for elderly people and underestimate BMI, not taking into account the muscle mass they have lost through the years. However, for the majority of us, BMI is a good general indicator of our healthy weight range and whether we are putting ourselves at risk.

You can crunch the numbers yourself by using this formula:

Weight in pounds/[height in inches]^2 x 703

You can also find calculators online, such as the one at *www.choosemyplate.gov/supertracker-tools/resources/bmi-calculator.html*.

Or you can use the chart on pages 114 and 115 to easily find your BMI. To use this BMI chart, locate your height in the left-hand column and follow the row across that height to find your weight. Follow that column of the weight up to the top to locate your BMI.

Now that you know your BMI, what exactly does it mean? Healthy weight is a range, and not one single number. The following will show you what range you fall into and what your BMI means for you.

BMI	Weight
Below 18.5	Underweight
18.5 to 24.9	Healthy Weight
25.0 to 29.9	Overweight
Over 30.0	Obese

Your Nutrition Solution Tidbit: BMIs for children and adolescents are slightly different. Because they are continually growing, their BMI is instead plotted on a growth chart. The percentile indicates the relative position of a child's BMI compared to that of children of the same gender and age.

Why Does My Body Shape Matter?

BMI is only one factor in assessing your weight. For an accurate assessment of weight related to health it is also important to look at *where* you store fat. The shape of our bodies, or where we store that excess fat, is compared to fruit—either an apple or a pear. If you are shaped more like an apple, meaning you store and carry the majority of your fat in the stomach area and around your waist, you are at a higher risk for certain health problems such as cardiovascular disease, high blood pressure, type 2 diabetes, and certain types of cancer. If you are shaped more like a pear, meaning you store and carry the majority of your fat below the waist, in your hips, buttocks, and thighs, your shape does not put you at as much of a health risk.

							Weight in Pounds										
BMI	19	20	21	22	23	24	25	26	27	28	29	30	31	32	33	34	35
Height																	
4'10"	91	96	100	105	110	115	119	124	129	134	138	143	148	153	158	162	167
4'11"	94	99	104	109	114	119	124	128	133	138	143	148	153	158	163	168	173
5'	97	102	107	112	118	123	128	133	138	143	148	153	158	163	168	174	179
5'1"	100	106	111	116	122	127	132	137	143	148	153	158	164	169	174	180	185
5'2"	104	109	115	120	126	131	136	142	147	153	158	164	169	175	180	186	191
5'3"	107	113	118	124	130	135	141	146	152	158	163	169	175	180	186	191	197
5'4"	110	116	122	128	134	140	145	151	157	163	169	174	180	186	192	197	204
5'5"	114	120	126	132	138	144	150	156	162	168	174	180	186	192	198	204	210
5'6"	118	124	130	136	142	148	155	161	167	173	179	186	192	198	204	210	216
5'7"	121	127	134	140	146	153	159	166	172	178	185	191	198	204	211	217	223

5'8"	125	131	138	144	151	158	164	171	177	184	190	197	203	210	216	223	230
5'9"	128	135	142	149	155	162	169	176	182	189	196	203	209	216	223	230	236
5'10"	132	139	146	153	160	167	174	181	188	195	202	209	216	222	229	236	243
5'11"	136	143	150	157	165	172	179	186	193	200	208	215	222	229	236	243	250
6'	140	147	154	162	169	177	184	191	199	206	213	221	228	235	242	250	258
6'1"	144	151	159	166	174	182	189	197	204	212	219	227	235	242	250	257	265
6'2"	148	155	163	171	179	186	194	202	210	218	225	233	241	249	256	264	272
6'3"	152	160	168	176	184	192	200	208	216	224	232	240	248	256	264	272	279
6'4"	156	164	172	180	189	197	205	213	221	230	238	246	254	263	271	279	287
	Healthy Weight						Overweight					Obese					

Source: Evidence Report of Clinical Guidelines on the Identification, Evaluation, and Treatment of Overweight and Obesity in Adults, 1998. NIH/National Heart, Lung, and Blood Institute (NHLBI). Check out www.nhlbi.nih.gov/guidelines/obesity/bmi_tbl.htm for additional heights and weights.

But this doesn't mean you don't need to drop that extra weight!

Most of us are painfully aware of where we store every little bit of fat, so you shouldn't have much problem figuring out what fruit you resemble. But if you just can't decide whether you look more like an apple or a pear you can use your waist-to-hip ratio. Your waist-to-hip ratio can help determine, in a more scientific way, if the location of your body fat is putting you at greater risk for health problems related to your weight.

Follow these steps to figure out your waist-to-hip ratio:

1. Stand relaxed. Measure your waist at its smallest point (just above your hip bone), without sucking in your stomach or pulling the tape measure too tight.

2. Measure your hips by measuring the largest part of your buttocks and hips.

3. Divide your waist measurement by your hip measurement.

4. If this number is close to or more than 1.0, you would be considered an apple shape.

5. If this number is considerably less than 1.0, you would be considered a pear shape.

Why is this important to you? The more body fat you carry in the stomach and waist area the more at risk you are for acid reflux and GERD. And if you already have acid reflux and GERD, body fat in these areas will only worsen your symptoms. So it seems that where you store fat on your body may be just as important, or maybe even more important, than how much excess body fat you have.

> **Your Nutrition Tidbit:** Your body shape, whether apple or pear, can be an inherited gene. In other words, where you carry body fat can be something that is passed down through your family tree, and something you don't have a whole lot of control over. But if you realize you are an apple shape, you can take extra precautions now to keep your weight healthy and your body fat down so that you don't deal with GERD down the road. If you are more of an apple shape with excess body weight and you experience acid reflux, be assured that losing weight will be a big positive step toward reducing your current symptoms as well as future damage.

Steps to Weight Loss

There are so many necessary reasons to reach a healthy weight, and if you are reading this book then trying to control your acid reflux and/or GERD successfully for the long term is probably at the top of your list. If you have a ways to go to get to your healthy weight range, take heart in knowing that a little bit can go a long way. If you are on the overweight side of the coin, losing just 5 to 10 percent of your current weight can sometimes be just the ticket to improve your health and to begin improving your symptoms of acid reflux. But you can't stop there! Reaching your healthy weight once and for all will not only help to bring your acid reflux under control, but it will also most likely end up helping in ways you never even considered.

If you are like most people, you want to lose weight the quickest and easiest way possible. Who doesn't?! But resist the urge to sign up for fad diets that promise quick and easy weight loss. These types of diets usually revolve around deprivation of some type and that can easily deplete your body's stores of essential nutrients. Furthermore, losing weight too quickly is usually the weight loss that never sticks. Also steer clear of liquid diets, diet pills, or diet supplements that promise that tempting quick fix. Slow and steady wins the race to long-lasting weight loss, better health, and improved GERD symptoms. Losing just 1 to 2 pounds per week is a safe and effective goal. The ultimate goal should not only be to get rid of those nasty acid reflux symptoms but also to lose the weight and keep it off for good!

It doesn't take as much change as you think to begin losing weight. You can do it safely by adding or subtracting as little as 250 to 500 calories per day. That can be as simple as eliminating a regular can of soft drink and that mid-day candy bar, neither of which are doing your acid reflux any good anyhow! There is no need to drastically slash your food intake all at one time or change your entire diet around. Instead, make changes and cut back slowly. Making healthier choices by eliminating unhealthy foods and replacing them with healthier foods will automatically cut calorie intake. As you lose weight and your body becomes accustomed to this new calorie level, which you might notice by experiencing a weight plateau, it may be time to make a few more changes and cut back a bit more. The idea is that for permanent weight loss you want to lose weight slowly, steadily, and in a healthy manner.

The key is to worry less about every little calorie and concentrate more in general on eating nutrient-rich foods that make calories count while still keeping an eye on your portion sizes, which will keep control of your calorie intake. This will ensure that even though you are trying to lose weight you will still be getting all the essential nutrients your body needs for good health. It is time to change bad habits into good ones, and that goes for eating as well as exercise. Here are just a few strategies that may help you begin losing weight in a way that is healthy and that lowers your risk of symptoms from acid reflux:

- ℵ Your first order of business should be to think hard about your true reasons for wanting to lose weight. Because you are reading this book it is a good bet that reducing acid reflux symptoms without the need for medications will be somewhere on that list. Knowing exactly what will motivate you and keep you committed to your goals is what will ultimately make you successful in your endeavor! To stay committed to your motivations, write them down and look at them when you need that extra boost to keep you going.

- ℵ You need to set goals. Set both short-term and long-term goals. Short-term goals are essential to keep you going on the journey to reach your long-term goal of a healthy weight. Your goals need to be realistic, specific, and measurable. Write them down, along with your motivations, so you always know what you are working toward. Don't expect to change *all* of your bad habits, or the habits that have caused that extra weight gain, all at one time. Work on changing habits a few at a time. Once you have mastered one goal, move on to the next.

⋈ Keep a daily food diary that includes what you eat, when you eat, and how much you eat. Write it down or find a free online food diary such as the Food Tracker on ChooseMyPlate.gov. Review your food diary frequently so that you can pinpoint and work on problem areas. Keeping a food diary will help to keep you compliant and on track.

⋈ Get in the habit of being aware of every food and beverage you put in your mouth. Make yourself accountable for what you eat and the way you live your life. For the most part you should not eat for reasons other than true hunger and for properly fueling your body.

⋈ Do *not* skip meals—and that includes breakfast. You won't save calories. Skipping a meal will lead to eating more at the next meal than you should, and/or will cause uncontrolled snacking throughout the day. Both of these behaviors will pack on more calories than you need.

⋈ Stick to a well-balanced and healthy eating routine. Healthier choices usually mean fewer calories, less fat, less sodium, and more nutritional value. The USDA's Dietary Guidelines for Americans (*www. health.gov/dietaryguidelines/2010.asp*) can provide you with information on good dietary habits.

❧ Cut back or cut out your junk foods such as candy, cookies, cake, pies, other sweets, soft drinks, fast foods, and chips. Occasional consumption of these foods is okay, but frequently eating them causes weight gain.

❧ Plan your healthy meals and snacks ahead of time so that you are always prepared.

❧ Practice and become aware of portion control. Sticking to more moderate portion sizes will not only help with weight loss, but not overeating will also minimize abdominal pressure and help reduce acid reflux. So keep your portions smaller and don't overfill your stomach. Eat until you are comfortable, not stuffed.

❧ Avoid eating in front of the television (especially late-night snacks) or computer or while doing other activities that keep you from paying attention to how much you are eating. Skipping those late-night snacks will cut unneeded calories from your day as well as help reduce the incidence of acid reflux at night that can make sleeping difficult.

❧ Get in the habit of slowing yourself down while eating. It takes a good 20 minutes for your brain to get the message that you are full. Eating too quickly leads to overeating, which can lead to excess weight as well as acid reflux. Eating slower can result in eating less and saving yourself the pain of heartburn.

❧ Use a smaller-sized plate to dish up your food. It will help to keep your portions and calories under control and make you feel that you are getting a full plate of food. Just don't go back for seconds!

❧ Plan and prepare more meals at home to keep from eating out too often. You don't have to be a chef to do this. Invest in some healthy cookbooks, check online, or share recipes with friends. Restaurant meals tend to be higher in calories, and it can sometimes be too tempting to make the right choices when eating out. Don't deprive yourself of eating out, but make it an occasional outing instead of a regular habit and work on making better choices when you do eat out.

❧ Learn how to read and use food labels to your advantage. (See *www.choosemyplate.gov/supertrack-er-tools/food-labeling.html*.) Food labels help you choose foods that best fit into your goals. They will help provide you with a good measurement of portion sizes and calorie intake.

❧ Check out the USDA's ChooseMyPlate.gov site to explore all of the information and hands-on tools that can help you lose weight sensibly and at the same time teach you what good nutrition really means.

❧ Incorporate some type of physical activity most days of the week. Overweight and obesity is a direct result of an imbalance between the calories you take in and the calories you burn. It is just that simple. The more active you are the more calories you will burn. Something as simple as walking can be a great start.

- Drink plenty of water throughout each day. Staying properly hydrated is essential to digestion and the fat-burning process. Keep in mind that it is best to drink liquids between meals instead of with meals to minimize symptoms of acid reflux.

- If you feel you need more personal guidance (and many people do), turn to a Registered Dietitian (RD) or Registered Dietitian Nutritionist (RDN) who can educate, guide, motivate, and keep you on track to future success. You can check out *www.eatright.org* to find a dietitian in your area.

- While you are on your way to weight loss success remember to avoid foods and beverages that may trigger your heartburn. Once you have lost weight you may find you can eat some of the foods that once gave you trouble. You can introduce these foods back in your diet one by one, after you have reached your healthy goal weight.

These simple tips and changes can help you improve your health, lose weight, and reduce acid reflux. It is all about lifestyle change and making permanent changes that you can and will stick with for life. Once you begin to lose weight and feel your acid reflux symptoms getting better you will be motivated to push ahead and finish your journey.

Your Nutrition Solution Tidbit: About 3,500 calories add up to one pound. Therefore, to lose one pound per week you need to split up a deficit of 3,500 calories over a week's time.

Deducting 500 calories per day should result in a one-pound-per-week weight loss.

Step 4: Identify Your Trigger Foods

So far we have learned that there are numerous factors that can trigger acid reflux, including poor lifestyle habits and dietary intake, excess weight, pregnancy, medical problems such as hiatal hernia, and even some medications. We also know that everyone does not have the same triggers. The goal is to find out what triggers *your* acid reflux and fix it so that you can live a life free of symptoms without being on medications that are not meant to be taken for long periods of time. If nothing we have discussed so far sounds like your trigger then maybe you need to dig a bit deeper.

Specific foods can be a trigger for acid reflux in some people. Of course there are the usual lists of common "bad" foods to stay away from, but those are for the general population and don't always pertain to each individual (these will be discussed in Chapter 4). However, if you don't know your triggers, it is a good place to start. Pinpointing your food triggers so that you can avoid them and your symptoms of GERD may just be your best medicine for fighting your acid reflux, but it is not always easy to find out what they are. Here are a few ways to identify these foods so that you can get to the root of your problems.

Personal Trigger Journal

One way to identify your trigger foods is to keep a personal food diary or trigger journal. This can be as easy as a notebook you carry with you or as complex as a spread-sheet you create on your computer. Keeping a journal can help you and your doctor determine what may be caus-ing the majority of your symptoms. Your trigger journal should include the foods and beverages you consume and how much, what time you eat them, what you did physi-cally before and after, and what type of symptoms you did or did not experience. There is no one specific diet for GERD that will work for all people. The only one that will work for you is one that is personally created around the food and activities that aggravate *your* reflux.

Your trigger journal might look something like the one on the following page.

You need to continue with your journal faithfully, ev-ery day, for at least a few weeks. The longer you continue with it the larger variety of foods, beverages, and activi-ties you will be able to experiment with, which gives you more data on which to base your conclusions. Once you have given yourself enough time to gather information, look over it and note when you experienced symptoms. Look down the columns and try to find similarities in the data you have collected. For example, you may want to question regular coffee if you had one cup for breakfast and one cup in the afternoon every day and each time you drank the coffee, regardless of what else you ate, you experienced heartburn. However, if you experience heart-burn only in the morning after coffee but not in the after-noon, you may need to look a bit more closely. Maybe you had orange juice with breakfast and that is the culprit. As you look through your journal, identify and write down all

My Trigger Journal				
Food/ Beverage Consumed	How Much	Time of Day	Activities Before, During, and After	Symptoms and Time of Day
Hardboiled egg	1			
Orange Juice	1/2 cup			
Regular coffee with cream and sugar	2 cups	8:15 a.m. (breakfast)	Watched TV Walked 45 mins.	Mild heartburn about 15 mins. after eating
Whole-wheat toast with butter and jelly	2 slices, 1 tsp jelly			

of the foods and/or beverages you suspect as triggers. This will begin to provide you with a good start toward eliminating those things that cause your symptoms. It may take some work, and you still may be left scratching your head at certain times, but continue with your journal. Much of identifying triggers with a food journal involves trial and error. Avoid the triggers you identify and see if your symptoms improve. You can speak with your doctor about getting a registered dietitian (RD) or registered dietitian nutritionist (RDN) involved in the process to help you identify problem foods and to also help guide you on what foods to use to replace those eliminated trigger foods if needed.

Elimination Diet

Another way to discover your personal triggers for acid reflux is to start with a clean slate. This can be done by eliminating *all* foods from your diet that are known as common triggers for heartburn (you can find these foods and beverages in Chapter 4). Then you can begin to add these foods and beverages back into your diet one by one to find out which ones are causing you the most problems. The best way to do this is to keep a food journal once you have eliminated those possible triggers. As you add foods and beverages back into your diet give each one at least a week to see if patterns develop with that food or beverage. If there is nothing noted, that food can go on your safe list, but if you notice a pattern of heartburn each time that food or beverage is consumed consider that food one of your triggers and eliminate it from you diet. This process, as with a trigger journal, can be time consuming, and you will go through some trial and error, but it will help you to start weeding out the foods and beverages—and only those foods and beverages—that cause problems for you. There's no sense in eliminating all common foods that trigger heartburn if they don't cause *your* symptoms. As with keeping a food journal, if you decide to go this route to identify your trigger foods, it is best to seek the help of an RD or RDN to guide you properly through the process.

MRT (Mediator Release Testing) and LEAP (Lifestyle, Eating, and Performance)

As we discussed in Chapter 1, science has confirmed a link between food allergies/sensitivities and symptoms of acid reflux. If you can find out which foods you are allergic or sensitive to you may be able to find the root of your acid reflux problems. So how do you find out? One way is an MRT, or Mediator Release Test. An MRT is a blood test that measures your immune reaction or sensitivity to a host of foods and chemicals. The results identify a safe list of foods to eat that will not trigger acid reflux, improving not only your symptoms but also any possible damage done to the GI tract. MRT has been shown to have the highest level of accuracy of any food-sensitivity blood test. This type of testing can often help to identify culprits that a person cannot figure out any other way. The hub of the immune system is essentially the gut, and when a person consumes a food that she has a reaction or a sensitivity to, her immune system sends out chemical mediators such as histamine, cytokines, and prostaglandins, which can produce damaging effects on body tissues and cause the development of symptoms. Depending on the types of mediators released, different areas of the body are affected. For example, for some people, consuming a trigger food will cause migraines; for others, arthritis; and for others still, acid reflux. Some people will deal with a myriad of symptoms, whereas others will experience one single symptom, such as reflux. Identifying the harmful substance is the first step toward improving your reflux symptoms related to food sensitivities. The next step involves following an individualized LEAP eating plan.

Many of you have probably never heard of LEAP (Lifestyle, Eating, and Performance), but this could be your answer to finding out once and for all what foods and/or beverages are truly triggering your GERD. LEAP is an effective protocol that combines the Mediator Release Test (MRT) with the professional skills of a Certified LEAP Therapist (CLT). The CLT is able to produce a patient-specific anti-inflammatory diet dependent on the results of your MRT to reduce inflammation and therefore reduce symptoms of health issues such as GERD. The two go hand-in-hand and have had substantial results for many individuals. A Certified LEAP Therapist, usually a dietitian, has received advanced clinical training in adverse food reactions, including food allergies, food sensitivities, and food intolerance. They know exactly how to assist clients with their LEAP Diet Protocols, which are based directly on the results of their MRT blood test.

Most people who have MRT testing done along with counseling from a CLT have experienced significant improvement within the first 10 days, with symptoms continuing to improve throughout the next 4 to 6 weeks. Many people experience complete symptom resolution once their triggers are identified and eliminated, depending on how closely they follow their LEAP protocol, whether they have underlying conditions involved, and to which degree food sensitivity plays a role in your condition. In fact, not only will you possibly be able to resolve your acid reflux symptoms, but you may be able to resolve other symptoms and health issues as well.

If you are interested in LEAP and MRT testing visit *http://nowleap.com* or call 1-888-Now-LEAP (toll free). In addition, there is a list of RDs and RDNs in the Resource section of this book to help get you started. Many CLTs will counsel via phone, so you don't even need to be in the same area. This process is definitely more than just being tested! Most people who are tested without counseling from a CLT do not do nearly as well. Talk to your doctor about being tested, and if you decide it is right for you, do it the correct way and partner with a LEAP Therapist. What you do with the test results is the most important part of the process.

Step 5: Practice Alternative Therapies

We have talked about food as a main trigger for acid reflux, but there are also other triggers, such as stress. Stress can cause the upper sphincter or the LES to relax (even though *you* are not relaxed!) and the bottom one to tighten, causing gastric juices to travel back up the esophagus and cause acid reflux. Stress is not a sole cause of GERD but it can make your symptoms to worsen and occur more frequently. Not only can stress lead to heartburn, but it can also cause you to gobble up your trigger foods without thinking about it! In addition to changing lifestyle and eating habits to manage acid reflux it is important to learn how to manage your stress.

Relaxation Therapies

Utilizing different relaxation therapies to calm stress and anxiety may help to reduce symptoms and frequency of GERD. Techniques include yoga, which has a calming effect that can reduce stress levels. Choose a type of yoga that involves relaxation, and choose a time to do your yoga when you don't have a full stomach.

Acupuncture is a relaxation therapy that involves inserting thin needles into specific points on your body. This can focus on specific areas such as the GI tract. Another good therapy is Reiki, which means *spiritually guided life energy*, or, more commonly, *universal life energy*. Reiki treatments are based on the channeling and balancing of positive energy within the body, through a practitioner, to promote overall health and healing. Reiki therapy sends the body into a deep state of relaxation, which is said to unlock the body's own healing powers. Whether these relaxation therapies are for you or not is up to you and your doctor.

Exercise/Physical Activity

If the more alternative therapies are not your bag then you can always opt for plain old exercise to help you relax and feel your best. Exercise can help you lose weight (which can be directly related to acid reflux), maintain a healthy weight, relieve stress, boost your mood, increase self-esteem, improve sleep, and decrease your risk for a number of health issues. The key when you have acid reflux or GERD is *moderate* exercise. For some people, vigorous exercise such as running can agitate their acid reflux; however, incorporating regular moderate, low-impact exercises such as walking or biking can be very beneficial. It is best to wait at least two hours after eating to work out. The most important factor about exercise and staying active is to find something that you enjoy so that you are likely to stick with it and perform it on a regular basis. If you are currently a couch potato or an occasional exerciser at most, start slow and work your way up. If you are really not sure where to start, walking is always a good choice. Always talk to your doctor first before staring an exercise routine.

According to the Dietary Guidelines for Americans, adults aged 18 to 64 years should do at least 2 hours and 30 minutes (or 150 minutes) each week of aerobic activity at a moderate level, or 1 hour and 15 minutes (or 75 minutes) each week of aerobic physical activity at a vigorous level. Being active five or more hours weekly can provide even more health benefits. Spreading your exercise over at least three days is suggested. Each activity should be done for at least 10 minutes at a time. Adults should also engage in resistance/strength-training activities such as push-ups, sit-ups, or weight-lifting at least two days per week.

Here are some brief descriptions of each type of exercise.

> א Aerobic Activity: The word *aerobic* literally means "with air." Therefore, in aerobic exercise your muscles require an increased supply of oxygen. Aerobic activity is also known as cardio activity because it also speeds your heart rate and improves your lung and heart fitness. Examples of these activities that would be best for those with GERD include brisk walking, swimming, and biking.

א **Resistance/Strength Training:** This type of activity helps to build and maintain muscles and bones by working them against gravity. Strength training is used for improving muscle strength and tone. In men, it will increase muscle size, and for women it usually means more tone without significant muscle size increase. This can include using free weights such as dumbbells and/or weight machines or stretch bands for resistance training.

א **Warm-up/Stretching/Balance Activities:** These types of activities can help to improve physical stability and flexibility, which can help reduce the risk for injuries and help you to move around easier. The best time to stretch, to prevent injury, is when your muscles are already warmed up. Try to hold each stretch for at least 15 seconds, and *never* bounce. Stretch to the point of mild tension, and not pain.

Exercise is not the only way to burn calories and stay more physically active. In addition to exercise it is essential to keep yourself moving throughout the day and increasing your activities of daily living. The more you move your body, the better! Here are some easy ideas you can start implementing in your daily life right now.

א Take an elevator instead of the stairs.

א Park at the far end of the parking lot for a longer walk, if it is safe.

א Forget the drive-thru at the bank; park and walk in.

- If you have a sit-down job, get up every 30 minutes or less and move around.

- Play actively with your kids instead of watching from the sidelines.

- Take the dog for regular walks.

- Wash your car yourself instead of taking it to the car wash.

- While on the phone walk around the house instead of sitting on the couch.

Your Nutrition Solution Tidbit: Drink plenty of water before, during, and after exercise to help you and your muscles stay well hydrated. Avoid sports drinks, which can aggravate acid reflux.

chapter 4

10 foods to avoid and 10 foods to include

Food plays a huge role in causing or irritating acid re-flux, and not everyone has the same food triggers for their symptoms. However, certain foods and beverages *tend* to trigger symptoms in a good majority of people. Luckily, on the other side of the coin, certain other foods are commonly known to *benefit* those who suffer from acid reflux. We'll start with the 10 most common foods to avoid.

10 Common Culprits

If you don't know what your food triggers are, this list is a good place to start. As we discussed in Chapter 3, try eliminating these first and then add them back one by one to see which, if any, cause problems for you. The key is not to rule out entire groups of foods, such as fruits and vegetables, because you aren't sure which ones bother you. You need to find your triggers and avoid those foods only.

1. **Citrus fruits and tomatoes.** As important as fruits and veggies are to good health, there are a few that seem to commonly cause or worsen GERD symptoms in many people. The National Institutes of Health (NIH) has identified citrus fruits such as oranges, lemons, limes, and grapefruit, along with tomatoes and tomato-based products, as major offenders of acid reflux. These foods are very acidic and are likely to cause heartburn in those who are prone to it, especially if consumed on an empty stomach. Vegetables such as broccoli, cauliflower, cabbage, and Brussels sprouts can be gassy and therefore cause heartburn symptoms in those with GERD, so experiment to see what you can tolerate.

2. **Raw garlic and onions.** Some spices are more likely to cause heartburn than others. These include cloves, mint, mustard seed, nutmeg, and fresh garlic. Garlic is widely used but known to possibly cause upset stomach and bloating in some people. In addition to garlic, many people who experience heartburn do not do well with raw onions. However, this pertains mostly to those who already

suffer from acid reflux. Symptoms don't normally increase in those who weren't frequent heartburn sufferers already.

3. **Coffee.** The jury still seems to be out on this one, but it is believed that coffee can relax the LES, causing reflux symptoms for some. Coffee is highly acidic and can stimulate the secretion of gastric acids. That may even go for decaffeinated coffee as well, suggesting that other components of coffee, besides caffeine, may contribute to its aggravating effects. In fact, decaffeinated coffee has been shown to raise gastric acids more than caffeinated coffee. Knowing your personal tolerance for coffee is your best bet. One piece of good news is that there are some brands of "low acid" coffees.

4. **High-fat and fried foods.** Foods that are high in fat may not be as high in acidity and therefore may not get as much press when it comes to heartburn, but they can take a toll on GERD sufferers. High-fat foods, whether they are greasy, fried, fast foods; cheese; a juicy Rib Eye steak; or yummy chicken wings; take more time and stomach acid to digest, which delays stomach emptying and can relax the LES. This in turn allows your stomach to increase acid production and become bloated, both of which will worsen acid reflux symptoms. Because we shouldn't be eating these types of saturated fats for good health anyway, choose leaner varieties such as skinless poultry, seafood, beans, lean cuts of red meat, and low-fat or fat-free dairy products. Unhealthy and dangerous trans fats have also been

connected to esophageal disease and should be extremely limited in any diet. Not only will these changes benefit your reflux, but they will improve your weight and your health as well. Triple bonus!

5. **Chocolate.** We all love chocolate, but unfortunately for some it can be a trigger for heartburn. Chocolate contains a chemical called methylxanthine that can relax the muscle between your esophagus and stomach, or the LES, allowing acid to flow back up into the esophagus. Chocolate also contains caffeine and other stimulants such as theobromine, is higher in fat, and contains cocoa, all of which can agitate reflux. Although healthwise dark chocolate is better for us it is still chocolate and not great for those who already suffer with acid reflux. With any luck, chocolate is not one of your trigger foods!

6. **Spicy foods.** Spicy or "hot" foods and spices such as chili powder, curry powder, hot sauce, and pepper are known to irritate the esophagus and cause symptoms of heartburn. Avoiding these types of foods and seasonings if you have GERD may help to prevent symptoms and reduce your risk of ulcerations.

7. **Peppermint.** Peppermint, a popular flavoring in gum, toothpaste, hard candy, and tea has long been used to soothe an upset stomach and aid in digestion. It is even used to treat headaches, skin irritations, anxiety, depression, nausea, and diarrhea, but for people with GERD it can make heartburn worse. Peppermint relaxes and soothes the LES, allowing gastric juices to reflux back up into

the esophagus, causing symptoms of heartburn. If you suffer with GERD you may want to avoid peppermint as well as peppermint-flavored teas.

8. **Caffeine.** Coffee, soft drinks, hot tea, iced tea, and other caffeinated foods and beverages are often big offenders. Caffeine-containing products can stimulate acid production and relax the LES, which can worsen acid reflux symptoms. You don't have to give up *all* of your coffee or other caffeinated beverages, but you do need to cut back and watch your portion sizes. If you guzzle coffee all day long, chances are you will end up with heartburn as a consequence. Better yet, try switching to something like chamomile tea or green tea that is lightly brewed. Cutting back on coffee and other caffeinated beverages may or may not help; this is something you will need to experiment with and see how much is too much for you. However, if you are a big coffee drinker it is probably a smart idea to cut back either way.

9. **Carbonated drinks.** Those little bubbles that seem so harmless in our favorite soft drink can often aggravate your reflux. They expand inside the stomach, which in turn increases pressure on the esophageal sphincter or LES, promoting symptoms of reflux such as heartburn. In addition, because the carbonation increases stomach pressure it tends to cause burping, which can cause the LES to open, again increasing your chances of acid reflux and heartburn. Soft drinks that are both carbonated and contain caffeine are even worse. Your best bet

is plain old water. Drinking a small glass of water at the end of meals may help to dilute stomach acids and reduce the risk of reflux. It can also help to soothe the burn of heartburn by washing stomach acids out of the esophagus. It won't get rid of it altogether, but it may help your symptoms a bit.

10. **Alcohol.** Wine, beer, and your favorite cocktail can turn happy hour sour, especially if you add it to a large meal. Most alcoholic beverages themselves are usually not very acidic, but alcohol tends to open and relax the LES, allowing the acid free passage back up into your esophagus. In addition, it stimulates production of stomach acid and makes the esophagus more sensitive to stomach acid. If you still want to enjoy an alcoholic beverage occasionally, these tricks may help:

   - Dilute your beverage with water or club soda.

   - Drink only moderate amounts.

   - Drink white wine instead of red. (Red tends to be more acidic, so it can cause problems for some.)

   - Avoid lying down after you have a drink.

   - Choose non-alcoholic beer or wine.

   - Keep track of which alcoholic beverages aggravate your heartburn the most, and avoid those.

   - Avoid using acidic mixers such as orange juice or caffeinated soft drinks.

11. If all alcohol seems to aggravate your heartburn it is best to avoid it altogether.

10 Potential Helpers

Just as there are foods that trigger heartburn, there are foods that can help you fight your heartburn. They all won't work for everyone, but you never know what might work for you. There are many possibilities, but we will just talk about 10 of the top beneficial foods. Keep in mind that some of these foods can also be a trigger food for you, so proceed with caution.

1. **Ginger.** Ginger or ginger root has been used for centuries as a spice and for medicinal purposes. This spice has anti-inflammatory properties and is known to be a treatment for stomach problems. It is claimed to be effective in absorbing stomach acid, which in turn can benefit GERD. You can steep raw ginger in hot water as a tea, add it to a smoothie, chew fresh ginger root, use it as a spice in cooking and baking, or take it in a capsule form following meals. Be careful of using too much, because this can actually cause heartburn.

2. **Almonds.** If you are a nut lover you will be happy to know that almonds, whether roasted, salted, or unsalted, can be effective in treating heartburn symptoms. Almonds are an alkaline-producing food and can help balance the pH in your GI tract, lowering the acid and helping to reduce heartburn. Pop three or four of those healthy nuts right after a meal or snack and chew them up well so that the oil is released from the almond. As a bonus, almonds are a good source of calcium and "healthy" fats—but they are also high in calories, so stick

to popping just a few. Additionally, because they are high in fat (even though it's the "good" fat), they also can cause heartburn in some, especially if eaten in large amounts.

3.   **Oatmeal.** Start your day with oatmeal instead of a greasy breakfast that includes foods like bacon and sausage, which can and probably will trigger your heartburn. Giving yourself heartburn with your first meal is not a good start to the day! Oatmeal is low in fat and high in fiber and can soothe your stomach—a much better way to start your day. Including higher-fiber foods in your daily diet can help naturally decrease your chances of experiencing acid reflux.

4.   **Bananas.** Besides being a nutritious fruit, bananas may have an antacid effect on your stomach and can also remove a particular type of bacteria linked to ulcer formation. Bananas have a naturally low acid content. Try incorporating a piece of banana shortly before a meal, with a meal, or shortly after a meal to see if it brings you any relief. You may also try eating a banana anytime during the day that you feel heartburn symptoms. Eat bananas at the right time: when they are under-ripe they have a higher acid content so make sure they are ripened and not too green on the outside.

5.   **Yogurt.** Yogurt can be beneficial for acid reflux because of the probiotics it contains. We discussed probiotics in Chapter 2, so we know that they are "friendly" bacteria that are present and essential for

a healthy digestive system. Eating yogurt is one of the best ways to consume probiotics as it contains live strains of these good bacteria. Eating yogurt with probiotics can help to restore and maintain the natural pH balance of the gut, which can help reduce the effects of acid reflux.

Your Nutrition Solution Tidbit: When choosing yogurt, opt for fat-free or low-fat varieties and be sure to check the label for "live and active cultures." Choose a yogurt that has plenty of protein, lower sugar content, and a boost of vitamin D. Get in the habit of adding a tablespoon of ground flaxseed when you eat your yogurt. This will add fiber as well as healthy omega-3 fats, which are both beneficial to acid reflux.

6. **Fennel and fennel seeds.** The fennel bulb is a vegetable that can be a great food to add for acid reflux. It may help to improve stomach function and contains a substance that may help to calm spasms in the digestive tract. Fennel contains health-benefiting nutrients such as antioxidants, dietary fiber, vitamins, and minerals. This crunchy veggie has a unique mild-licorice flavor. If you cut the white bottom part into thin slices it is great to add to salads. You can add it to chicken dishes and other recipes as well. Fennel seeds are also used for medicinal purposes as they contain disease-fighting antioxidant flavonoids such as quercetin and

kaempferol and are a rich source of dietary fiber as well as many vitamins and minerals. Essential oils found in fennel seeds aide the digestive system, which in turn can help with indigestion and symptoms of acid reflux. Fennel seeds can be found as either whole seeds or as a powder, though seeds are best. In addition, fennel has been known to help lower cholesterol, ease constipation, work as an anti-inflammatory, and moisturize a dry scalp.

7. **Seafood.** One of the best things you can do for acid reflux is to eat low-fat, high-protein meals. Seafood is a good staple to have in your diet because it rarely causes symptoms of acid reflux. Seafood is chock-full of healthy omega-3 fatty acids (some fish more than others), and is low in saturated "bad" fat and high in protein. Omega-3 fatty acids act as an anti-inflammatory and have countless health benefits. Try to include fish that is wild-caught versus fish that is farm-raised. Grill, bake, or broil your fish and seafood and refrain from adding creamy sauces or eating seafood that is breaded and deep-fried, which can add to reflux symptoms.

Your Nutrition Solution Tidbit: Although fish can be very healthy and essential to good health, fish oil supplements may trigger heartburn for some people. Fish oil supplements are a good way to get that extra boost of healthy omega-3 fats, especially for those who don't care for fish or other seafood. If you find that your supplement is causing heartburn, try taking your fish oil supplement with meals. Another solution may be to try and freeze your supplements before taking them. Also try starting out with a lower dose and slowly working your dosage up as your body and digestive system become accustomed to it. If none of these solutions work, speak with your doctor.

8. **Pineapple and papaya.** Both pineapple and papaya contain proteases, which are digestive enzymes that help to facilitate the breakdown of protein in foods we consume. Pineapple contains Bromelain, an enzyme that both aids digestion and reduces inflammation; papaya contains Papain, an enzyme that digests protein. Our body normally uses the enzyme pepsin to digest or breakdown protein, but pepsin is not very effective unless it is in a very acidic environment. Because most people with GERD are on a low-acid eating plan, digestion of proteins may become more difficult, resulting in reflux. Adding these two fruits to your diet may help to alleviate reflux caused by this problem. For the most benefits, choose pineapple that is raw or frozen.

9. **Parsley.** Most of us think of parsley as that useless but pretty garnish on a plate. But parsley is more than that. Parsley is recognized as an herb that can help settle the stomach, ease stomach irritation, and aid in digestion. So there is a reason you find it on your plate as a garnish so often in restaurants.

Parsley contains an amino acid called glutamine, which may have anti-inflammatory properties. Glutamine may help to reduce intestinal inflammation as well as acid reflux. Parsley may also help to neutralize acids in the stomach enough to produce an alkaline balance and prevent the occurrence of heartburn. This is one versatile and helpful herb. Try adding it to soups, salads, casseroles, potatoes, and other favorite recipes.

10. **Pistachios.** If you're nuts over pistachios you may be in luck. Pistachios are great for digestion and just so happen to be full of nutritional value and fiber. They are packed with vitamins B6, thiamin, manganese, and copper. Recent research points toward these nuts as having periodic properties, meaning they help to support higher levels of beneficial bacteria in your digestive tract. As far as nuts and calories go, pistachios are on the low end. The fiber in these nuts along with their healthy unsaturated fats help keep the digestive system running smoothly and acid reflux to a minimum.

Other At-Home Remedies

- **Apple cider vinegar.** We talked previously about low stomach acid being a possible cause of acid reflux. If your GERD is related to the problem of low stomach acid, consuming vinegar may help by increasing the acidity and promoting digestion. As with other home remedies, this theory is not scientifically proven, but many people swear by its effectiveness and deem it one of the better natural ways of getting rid of heartburn. It is recommended to mix about 2 teaspoons of apple cider vinegar with 8 ounces of water and drink it before meals or when heartburn strikes. It doesn't have the most pleasant taste, but you can try artisan vinegar, which may be more expensive but more palatable. You can even try mixing the vinegar with honey in tea or putting it on salads, on vegetables, or in smoothies. As a rule of thumb, if you find that the vinegar worsens your acid reflux symptoms, then low acidity is probably not the cause of your reflux. If you want to try vinegar on a regular basis speak with your doctor first.

- **Chewing gum.** Many of us love to chew gum, especially after we eat to freshen our breath, but how can that be a home remedy for heartburn? Research has found that chewing gum stimulates the production of saliva in our mouths, which acts as an acid buffer or a neutralizer for stomach acid, helping to relieve heartburn. In addition, chewing gum encourages more frequent swallowing, which can help clear irritating acid out of your esophagus more quickly and help protect that area. It is suggested to chew a piece of gum for 30 minutes after eating a meal. When you choose a pack of gum, choose one that is sugar-free, to protect your teeth, in a non-mint flavor, as peppermint and spearmint can relax the LES and worsen reflux symptoms.

- **Baking soda.** Sodium bicarbonate, more commonly known as baking soda, may be a good way to calm heartburn. Baking soda can be used as an antacid to treat heartburn, indigestion, and upset stomach. Because it is an alkaline substance it can help to neutralize stomach acids. With reduced acidity in the stomach, gastric juices are less likely to flow back up into the esophagus, thereby reducing heartburn and regurgitation in the chest and throat. Even if you still experience a bit of reflux after drinking the baking soda solution, your stomach contents will be less acidic and won't irritate the esophagus as badly. It isn't the tastiest concoction but it works fast. However, using baking soda for heartburn is only a natural remedy to use if you experience it on occasion. If you have GERD and/or deal with acid reflux frequently, then baking soda is not the way to go. It is very high in sodium, a little more than 600 mg per half-teaspoon, so it could cause side effects such as water retention, and if you already have issues with blood pressure, this would definitely not be the way to go on a regular basis. Most recommendations for baking soda are to dilute half a teaspoon in a 4-ounce glass of water and not to use more than 3 tablespoons in a 24-hour period. It is important not to drink the mixture until all of the powder is completely dissolved and not to drink it if your stomach is overly full with food and/or liquids. Ask your doctor before trying this home remedy.

- **Aloe vera juice.** Aloe is a plant that is used to soothe everything from burns to stomach aches. Juice from the plant is believed to reduce inflammation, including that in the esophagus and the stomach. When using aloe vera juice be sure to use only products that are specifically made for internal use. Aloe gel taken directly from the plant should not be used for internal consumption. The suggested amount to drink is typically a quarter-cup approximately 20 minutes before a meal. You can purchase aloe vera juice in many health food or natural food stores as well as online. It is crucial to avoid aloe juice products that contain aloe latex, aloin, and/or aloe-emoin compounds, which can be powerful laxatives and cause additional problems.

Your Nutrition Solution Tidbit: If you have diabetes and use a glucose-lowering medication to control your blood sugar levels, you should avoid using aloe vera juice, as some studies suggest it can lower blood glucose (sugar) levels. Talk to your doctor first.

❧ **Honey.** Just a spoonful of honey may make the acid go back down. Honey's thick consistency acts as a soothing coating on the walls of the esophagus to help diminish the burning caused by reflux. The thickness of honey can also help prevent additional acid from coming back up. Honey has significant antibacterial properties that work against pathogens that are commonly found in gastric and skin ulcers. In addition, honey may have anti-inflammatory properties. How you take honey for acid reflux is key. It is recommended to take just a small spoonful 20 minutes before eating a meal and/or bedtime and not to drink any liquids between taking the honey and eating. Some also recommend mixing about 2 teaspoons of apple cider vinegar and 2 teaspoons of honey into a cup of warm water for a boost of acid reflux protection. Honey can also help those who deal with a chronic cough due to acid reflux.

Your Nutrition Solution Tidbit: For treating acid reflux, natural or organic honey works fine as well as local bought honey. However, there is another type of honey called *manuka* honey that has been shown to work even better on reflux and other digestive issues. This type of honey is native to New Zealand but you can find it in the United States. Manuka honey is considered medical grade and its antibacterial and healing properties have been researched extensively to show that it is superior to that of regular natural honey. It is much more expensive than regular store-bought honey, but the costmay be worth it.

✗ **Milk.** Drinking a glass of milk is probably the oldest remedy for heartburn in the book. The truth is that it most likely will help temporarily by buffering stomach acids. However, keep in mind that fat can stimulate the stomach to produce more acid, so if you are going to gulp a glass of milk for heartburn make sure it is fat-free or at the least low-fat. Following the popular suggestion of drinking a glass of milk before bedtime, even if it is fat-free, is discouraged. Eating or drinking anything right before bedtime and before lying down can stimulate acid reflux. For some people milk can even be a trigger. If milk is one of your triggers it is important to seek out comparable alternatives so you don't miss out on the essential nutrients that milk provides. Try drinking soy milk, almond milk, or rice milk as an alternative to cow's milk.

chapter 5

menu-planning and shopping guide

Now that you have learned the best way to eat for acid reflux and GERD it is time to get out there and put your plan into action by preparing menus and going grocery shopping. Each person's shopping list will of course be unique, because it will depend on one's personal trigger foods. However, I can give you general tips about menu planning and navigating the supermarket (including how to read labels) that will help everyone.

Menu-Planning Tips

The best way to make your life easier and free yourself from frequent heartburn is to plan ahead! Write out your menus for the week so that you can plan all your meals, snacks, and beverages around the general trigger foods as well as your own personal triggers. To begin planning you need to ask yourself where and when you will be eating in the next week and how much time you will have to cook. The more prepared you are the less likely you will be to eat out, eat on the run, or grab something you shouldn't— all of which can get you in trouble with heartburn.

Once your meals are planned, you can then create your shopping list. This will help you to buy only what is on your list and not stray to foods that are not on your safe list and/or are not healthy.

When planning your menus keep these tips in mind:

- Avoid the top-offender foods we listed in Chapter 4 and throughout this book unless you know for sure they don't trigger your acid reflux.

- Avoid your own personal triggers. Not having foods in the house that you know will trigger heartburn will ensure you stay away from them and are not tempted.

- Plan for small meals more frequently instead of two or three large ones. You will need to plan not only meals but also healthy snacks that will keep you heartburn-free. Also plan for meals or snacks that need to be taken to work or school.

❧ Plan meals that are made with fresh foods instead of using boxed or instant foods, which are more processed and can lead to heartburn. The more processed foods are, the more likely they are to be higher in sugar, sodium, and fat, and lower in whole grains as well as vitamin, minerals, and other essential nutrients. Buy a few recipe books or look online for some healthy, easy, and tasty recipes the whole family will enjoy.

❧ Plan meals and snacks to include more fruits, vegetables, and whole grains.

❧ Consider trying a vegetarian meal at least once a week to help cut back on fat and add more fiber to your diet. Studies have found that people who eat a higher-fiber diet are less likely to have acid reflux symptoms.

❧ When planning your menus, add some of the foods that can benefit acid reflux, such as parsley, almonds, ginger, and fennel. Look up some new recipes that incorporate some of these foods and spices.

❧ Stick to planning low-fat meals that are baked, grilled, or broiled. Keep foods with creamy sauces and other fatty additions off the menu, and try substituting lower-fat options.

Instead of...	Use...
whole milk	low-fat or fat-free milk
ice cream	sherbet or low-fat frozen yogurt
sour cream	plain non-fat yogurt
cream cheese	reduced-fat or fat-free cream cheese
bacon or sausage	Canadian bacon or lean ham
oil-packed tuna	water-packed tuna
whole eggs	egg whites
cookies	graham crackers or ginger snaps
chips	"light" microwaved popcorn
mayonnaise	pureed avocado
regular ground beef	extra-lean ground beef or lean ground turkey
chicken legs	skinless chicken breast

❧ Be creative and come up with some yummy substitutions in your menus for the foods that bother you the most so that you don't feel you are being deprived.

❧ Be sure to plan not only what you are making for meals but also the timing of your meals. Remember that you want to leave a good two to three hours after eating dinner before going to bed.

Your Nutrition Solution Tidbit: If you are not one to sit down and write things out, grab your phone and find an app for that! There are plenty out there that make planning your shopping list easy and fun.

Navigating the Supermarket

Eating a diet that will benefit your acid reflux and your health starts as you wheel your cart down each isle at the grocery store. But before you even get to the parking lot, make sure you eat a healthy meal or snack. Going shopping hungry can be your worst enemy! Grocery stores can be tough, with all of the foods you can't have staring you in the face at each turn. Your number-one weapon is a well-thought-out and well-organized grocery list that follows the meal plan you developed for the week. Here are a few tips to arm yourself with the next time you go grocery shopping so that you are able to fill your list with the healthiest foods from each aisle.

The Fruits and Vegetables Section

The first section you will come to in most grocery stores is the fresh fruit and vegetable section. This section of the grocery store is probably the largest, and is the one you should spend most of your time in. Fruits and veggies make great healthy snacks. Fruit can even be a great substitute for dessert or whenever you have a sweet tooth. Here are some pointers to help you get the most from this section.

- When choosing fruits and vegetables, keep in mind the produce you can and can't have. If you are not yet sure what your personal trigger foods are, avoid the foods that commonly cause heartburn such as citrus fruits and tomatoes, and purchase produce that is generally safe, such as apples, bananas, grapes, melons, pears, green beans, zucchini, carrots, potatoes, yams, and leafy greens.

- Look for produce with the most color. The more colorful they are the more nutrients they contain.

- Choose a variety of fruits and vegetables on your safe list each time you shop. Variety is the spice of life, and the more variety you choose the more nutritional value you will get. Be adventurous and try something new. That is the only way to find out if it will trigger reflux—and if you'll like it! You will have to experiment with fruits and vegetables to establish your safe list, so continue to write them down so you know which ones agree with you and which ones don't. Your safe list will be much bigger than your trigger list.

- ⋊ Buy fruits and vegetables that are in season and locally grown. Organic versions are always a great idea but can also be costly.

- ⋊ Pre-cut fruits and vegetables are a great idea for the busy person.

- ⋊ Buy fresh, frozen, dried, and/or canned (in 100% juice) fruits and veggies so that you always have something on hand.

- ⋊ When buying fresh, buy only what you need so that you can eat it up before it goes bad.

- ⋊ Avoid buying frozen or canned vegetables that contain added fats such as sauces or butter.

The Dairy Section

The "Dairy Case" lining the perimeter of the grocery store is often filled with all types of foods—some in the dairy food group and some not. The dairy case usually includes foods such as milk and milk alternatives like soy-milk, yogurts, cheeses, sour cream, cream cheese, eggs, puddings, butter and margarine, and dips. Keep in mind that the dairy section is full of high-fat foods, especially those with saturated and trans fats, which can trigger acid reflux. Here are some tips to help you choose wisely:

- ⋊ Since we already know that high-fat foods are a heartburn trigger, stick with low-fat and fat-free versions throughout the dairy case.

- ⋊ Choose margarines that do not contain trans fats or partially hydrogenated oils. Better yet, opt for oils such as olive oil when possible.

⋈ If milk is a trigger for you—or even if it isn't—try something like almond milk, as almonds can actually help with reflux.

⋈ Include low-fat and fat-free yogurts with lower sugar content and "live active cultures," which we know can have a positive impact on reflux.

The Meats/Seafood Section

This area of the grocery store, again in the "fresh" perimeter of the store, includes fresh meats, seafood, and fish as well as the deli section. Meats, especially red meats, can contain high amounts of saturated fats and calories. The goal here is to choose more lean meats and fish to help prevent reflux.

⋈ Choose lean meat choices such as skinless white-meat poultry, fish (wild caught), pork loin and tenderloin, top sirloin steak, eye of round roast, sirloin tip side steak, top round roast and steak, bottom round roast and steak, flank steak, chuck shoulder pot roast and steak, extra-lean ground beef (at least 90 percent or more lean), and extra-lean ground turkey. Cuts of meat are considered lean if they include the words "round" or "loin."

⋈ For lunch meats choose lean turkey, roast beef, lean ham, or chicken breast, and stay away from high-fat meats such as bologna and salami.

⋈ Opt for fewer red meats and more poultry and fish.

Your Nutrition Solution Tidbit: The American Heart Association recommends at least two servings of fish per week. Salmon is a great choice because it is widely available, affordable, and a good source of omega-3 fatty acids.

The Breads/Cereal/Rice/Pasta Sections

As you get to the center aisles of the grocery store you will encounter fewer fresh foods and more packaged and processed foods. This will include the breads, cereal, rice, and pasta sections, which offer you a great way to get your daily whole-grain and dietary fiber intake as well as other essential nutrients—if you make the right choices. Even if you suffer from GERD you can consume most starchy foods in these aisles. Specifically:

- Avoid refined foods such as white breads, regular pasta, white rice, and sugary cereals.

- Choose oatmeal, as it is not only a whole grain and high in fiber but also a benefit to those with GERD. Regular oatmeal is a better choice than instant because it is less processed, but even instant oatmeal is a whole grain. It makes a great breakfast or snack paired with fruit such as a banana or raisins and dried nuts such as almonds or walnuts.

- When choosing dry cereals, choose varieties that state "whole grain" and aim for at least 4 grams of fiber per serving and a lower sugar content.

- ⊠ Choose whole-wheat or whole-grain breads, cereals, and pasta and other high-fiber, whole-grain foods such as brown or wild rice.

- ⊠ Reading food labels is key in all sections but especially in this one. You will need to read labels to ensure you are choosing foods that are truly whole grains and have the fiber content you expect.

The Canned Food Sections

The canned food sections can include foods such as fruits, vegetables, tuna, beans, soups, and more. Keeping a variety of healthier canned goods on hand can ensure you always have something to reach for in a pinch. Choosing these foods, though not fresh, can still add to your required daily servings of certain foods groups. Canned foods can be just as nutritious if you make the right choices. For example:

- ⊠ Choose fruit that is canned in water or its own natural juices to keep sugar content down. Stay away from labels that state "in syrup."

- ⊠ Choose vegetables without added salt.

- ⊠ Choose tuna that is packed in water as opposed to oils.

- ⊠ Choose low-fat soups and try to stick with the broth-based soups that contain loads of vegetables.

- ⊠ Choose beans such as black, kidney, lentils, garbanzo, and navy, with no added salt, to add to soups, casseroles, whole-wheat pastas, and salads as an extra protein, nutrient, and fiber boost.

The Oils, Condiments, and Dressings Section

This can be a dangerous section, as it is filled with fats and sodium. But it just takes making some good choices to get through this isle in a healthy manner. Choices like:

- Choose healthy oils such as extra virgin olive oil and canola oil. But whether healthy or not, use them sparingly if you have GERD. A little bit can go a long way.

- If using margarines or spreads check the label for the words "partially hydrogenated" in the list of ingredients. These are the unhealthy trans fats and you should avoid these at all cost! There are many margarine spreads that are now made without trans fats.

- Steer clear of ketchup, hot sauce, salsa, and other condiments that may trigger reflux.

- Choose salad dressings that are more oil-based and are reduced-fat. Compare labels to choose ones lower in sodium and sugar. You best choice for salad dressing is a little extra virgin olive oil with apple cider vinegar, which may help with symptoms of reflux.

- Some sauces and condiments are quite high in sodium and sugar. Keep an eye on food labels, especially if you need to restrict your sodium.

- Try replacing regular mayonnaise with reduced-fat or fat-free versions, or try pre-packaged guacamole instead, if it isn't a trigger for you.

Your Nutrition Solution Tidbit: When choosing olive oil, opt for extra virgin, which is the purest form of olive oil and has the lowest acidity. This oil is great for dressings, drizzling on veggies, or brushing on breads. If you plan to cook with the oil it is best to go with virgin or light olive oil as they are better suited for heat. Always check dates because oils have a limited shelf life, and also choose a bottle from the back of the shelf, as light will tend to destroy the oil and its properties. Store it in a dark, cool, dry place once you get home.

The Frozen Foods Section

The frozen food section contains a large variety of foods such as vegetables, fruits, pizza, frozen entrees, breakfast foods such as pancakes and waffles, specialty items, breads, juices, and ice cream. Frozen foods such as fruits and vegetables are a convenient way to always have produce on hand, especially during the winter months. Here's how to choose the right items from this section.

- Be sure to read labels in the freezer section to help you choose the healthier versions of similar foods. For example, if you are choosing frozen breakfast foods opt for whole-grain waffles.

- When choosing veggies, choose ones that do not include sauces and butters. Many frozen vegetables come in ready-to-steam bags, which makes adding vegetables to meals even easier. Having frozen veggies on hand means you can always throw extra vegetables in soups, casseroles, pastas, and stews.

ン Frozen fruits are great for making smoothies or adding to your whole-grain waffles for breakfast or a snack. Choose frozen fruit without added sugar.

ン If choosing frozen meals/entrees you will need to read the nutrition facts panel. These meals are fine on occasion when you don't have time to cook, but don't rely on them regularly. In general, look for meals that include vegetables on your safe list, whole grains, and lean meat, fish, or poultry. Skip ones that include cream sauces, gravies, or fried foods and contain more than 600 mg of sodium. Don't assume these meals are healthy without first checking the label.

ン Choose low-fat ice cream or, better yet, low-fat frozen yogurt.

Using Food Labels to Help Your GERD

It is time to become a label reader so that you can determine, without guessing, whether a food is healthy and whether it will fit within the guidelines to reduce your acid reflux. The food label is full of information, including the Nutrition Facts Panel, Nutrient Content Claims, and Health Claims. All of these areas are regulated by the FDA and are meant to be used by the consumer to make informed choices.

The Nutrition Facts Panel

The "Nutrition Facts Panel" provides information about the nutrients people are most concerned about. This panel is the white rectangle on the back or side of food and beverage containers that lists all of the nutritional information. The Nutrition Facts Panel was mandated under the Nutrition Labeling and Education Act (NLEA) of 1990 and is based on recommendations from the Food and Drug Administration (FDA) and the U.S. Department of Agriculture (USDA). Understanding the information on this panel can help you to manage your health, your reflux, and your weight.

Nutrition Facts

Serving Size 1 cup (228g)
Servings Per Container about 2

Amount Per Serving

Calories 250	Calories from Fat 110

	% Daily Value*
Total Fat 12g	18%
Saturated Fat 3g	15%
Trans Fat 3g	
Cholesterol 30mg	10%
Sodium 470mg	20%
Total Carbohydrate 31g	10%
Dietary Fiber 0g	0%
Sugars 5g	
Proteins 5g	

Vitamin A	4%
Vitamin C	2%
Calcium	20%
Iron	4%

* Percent Daily Values are based on a 2,000 calorie diet. Your Daily Values may be higher or lower depending on your calorie needs:

	Calories:	2,000	2,500
Total Fat	Less than	65g	80g
Saturated Fat	Less than	20g	25g
Cholesterol	Less than	300mg	300mg
Sodium	Less than	2,400mg	2,400mg
Total Carbohydrate		300g	375g
Dietary Fiber		25g	30g

For educational purposes only. This label does not meet the labeling requirements described in 21 CFR 101.9.

You can use the Nutrition Facts Panel to your advantage by following a few simple tips.

Size It Up

One of the first parts of the label is the serving size, which is usually expressed in weight, volume, or number of units. Take a close look at the serving size and the servings per container. Ask yourself:

- How many calories are in a single serving?
- How many calories are in the entire package?
- How many servings do I plan to eat?

Keep in mind that *all* of the information on the Panel pertains to *one* single serving size. If you plan on eating two servings, then you need to double all of the information, including calories, fat, and %DV (Percent Daily Value). It's also important, when comparing calories and nutrients on the same food but between brands, to check whether the serving size is the same.

Your Nutrition Solution Tidbit: Many packages, including beverages, contain more than one serving. Don't fall into the trap of consuming an entire package assuming there is only one serving in it. That can add up to a lot more calories and fat then you bargained for.

Focus on Calories

Next on the label are calories and calories from fat. This is important for determining whether a food is appropriate for someone with acid reflux because most high-fat foods can trigger acid reflux. Because you are also focusing on either losing weight or maintaining a healthy weight, keep in mind that just because foods are fat-free that does not mean they're also calorie free! Check to see how many total calories the food contains and how many of those calories come from fat. For example, if a food has 300 calories per serving and 150 of those calories come from fat, then half of the calories in a single serving come from a fat source. Consider how the calories per serving will fit into your overall intake for the day. The key is to keep your calories in check as you manage your weight. Keep in mind that if you eat and drink more calories than you burn, you *will* gain weight.

In general, you can use the following guide to gauge the calories in a single product (based on a 2,000 calorie diet), but keep in mind that what really matters is the total calories you consume in a day and not what is in a single food.

LOW in calories = 40 calories per serving

Moderate in calories = 100 calories per serving

HIGH in calories = 400 calories or more per serving

Limit These Nutrients

The nutrients listed first on the label are the ones most Americans generally consume enough or too much of in their diet. These are nutrients to limit. They include total fat, saturated fat, trans fat, cholesterol, and sodium. It's not only important to know how much total fat is in a serving of a food but also what type of fat it is. Saturated and trans fats are the ones you want to limit.

Get Enough of These Nutrients

The nutrients listed next on the label are nutrients that most Americans *don't* get enough of in their diet, but need to. These include dietary fiber, vitamin A, vitamin C, calcium, and iron. Eating enough of these nutrients can help improve health and reduce the risk of some health conditions and diseases. Eating a diet high in fiber promotes a healthy digestive system, including a lower risk of GERD.

Figuring out Percent Daily Value

If you are not sure whether a food is high or low in the nutrients mentioned, the Percent Daily Value (%DV) is a tool on the label that can help you with that. Start with the footnote on the bottom of the label, which tells you that %DVs are based on a 2,000 calorie diet. This statement must appear on all food labels, even though it is the same on *all* labels and does not change from product to product like the rest of the information. This information is recommended dietary advice for all Americans and is not specific to the food product.

```
* Percent Daily Values are based on a 2,000 calorie diet.
  Your Daily Values may be higher or lower depending on
  your calorie needs:

                        Calories:  2,000      2,500
Total Fat               Less than  65g        80g
   Saturated Fat        Less than  20g        25g
Cholesterol             Less than  300mg      300mg
Sodium                  Less than  2,400mg    2,400mg
Total Carbohydrate                 300g       375g
   Dietary Fiber                   25g        30g
```

For educational purposes only. This label does not meet the labeling
requirements described in 21 CFR 101.9.

So, again, the recommendations for total fat, saturated fat, carbohydrates, and fiber are based on 2,000 calories. If you eat less than or more than these calorie levels you need to adjust the recommended dietary advice to fit your individual needs. Cholesterol and sodium recommendations are the same no matter what calorie level you are consuming. The following is a chart of how the Percent Daily Values need to be adjusted according to calorie level:

Adjusted Percent Daily Values for Specific Calorie Levels	
Calories	Adjusted %DV
1,200	60 percent
1,400	70 percent
1,600	80 percent

2,000	100 percent
2,200	110 percent
2,500	125 percent
2,800	140 percent
3,200	160 percent

Putting %DV to Use For You

Now that we know what the Daily Values are we can use them to determine Percent Daily Value (%DV), which will help you decide whether a food is high or low in a nutrient, and, ultimately if it is a smart food to choose. The %DV is listed to the right of most of the nutrients on the top part of the label.

To help you decide quickly, use this guide:

⌧ 5% DV or less is considered LOW for that nutrient

⌧ 20% DV or more is considered HIGH for that nutrient

Get enough of these nutrients *(The goal is to stay above 100% DV for each of these for the entire day)*:

⌧ Fiber

⌧ Vitamin A

⌧ Vitamin C

⌧ Calcium

⌧ Iron

Limit these nutrients *(The goal is to stay below 100%DV for each of these for the entire day)*:

- Total fat*
- Saturated fat
- Cholesterol
- Sodium

Stick to mostly polyunsaturated and monounsaturated fats, which are healthier fats.

You can use %DV not only to figure out if a food is high or low in a nutrient but also to compare products. You can easily compare one product or brand to a similar product to make the better choice. Just make sure when you compare that the serving sizes are similar. Serving sizes are kept generally consistent for similar types of foods to make comparing them easier for the consumer.

You can also use %DV to help you make dietary trade-offs with other foods throughout the day. This allows you to eat all of your favorite foods, on occasion, and fit them into a healthy diet. For instance, when one of your favorite foods is high in fat you can balance it with foods that are low in fat at other times of the day. But pay attention to how much you eat of that favorite food so that the total amount of fat for your day stays below the 100% DV.

One more way to use %DV is to help you distinguish one dietary claim from another, such as "light" versus "reduced fat." All you need to do is compare the %DVs for Total Fat in each of the foods to determine which one is higher or lower in that nutrient. This way there is no need to memorize all of the FDA's definitions of those claims.

Additional Nutrient Information

The label also provides %DVs for a few vitamins and minerals, including Vitamins A and C, calcium, and iron. You may see more on some labels, but you will at minimum always see these four nutrients. Use the %DV given so that you know how much one serving of a food contributes to the total amount you need per day.

The Daily Values used for these for nutrients are as follows:

- Vitamin A: 5,000 IU
- Vitamin C: 60 mg
- Calcium: 1,000 mg
- Iron: 18 mg*

These are general values; for certain populations some of these numbers may be higher or lower.

For example, if calcium in a food is listed as 25% DV, then one serving of that food will provide you with 25% of what you need for the day, or 250 mg.

Always check labels, and don't make assumptions. Just because yogurt is supposed to be a good calcium source, that doesn't mean every yogurt has the same amount of calcium. Before you buy, compare brands and choose the ones that have the most calcium and protein and the lowest sugar and fat content. Use the labels! They are on food products for consumers to use!

Your Nutrition Solution Tidbit: %DVs for trans fats, sugar, and protein have yet not been

established. However, you can still compare total amounts between brands to pick the better
product.

Putting It All Together

Once you have checked out all the parts of the food
label you need to ask yourself if this particular food is a
smart choice. Does it fit into a healthy diet, into your
weight management plan, and, most importantly, will it
cause you reflux? Ask these questions to find out:

⋈ Is one serving size enough for me, or do I need to
double or triple the calories, fat, and other nutrients on the label?

⋈ Are the calories per serving low, moderate, or
high? How many calories will be in the actual
amount I eat?

⋈ Are the nutrients that I need to limit low, and are
the nutrients I need more of high?

⋈ Is this food too high in fat, especially saturated
and trans fats?

⋈ Will this food provide me with some needed
fiber?

⋈ Have I compared the label on this product to
other brands of the same thing to ensure I am
getting the most bang for my buck? Should I look
for an alternative?

How you answer these questions will depend on your
calorie intake; whether you are trying to lose, maintain,

or gain weight; whether you might have specific nutritional needs; and which foods trigger your reflux the most. The bottom line is that food labels enable you to compare foods based on key ingredients and therefore make better choices. Food labels allow you to include your favorite foods occasionally, even if they are not always the smartest choices, while still you stick to your healthy eating plan and goals. Use the Nutrition Facts Panel to make your food choices easier and healthier!

Nutrient Content Claims on Food Labels

Even if you don't have time to read each and every food label, something known as Nutrient Content Claims, or NCCs, can help you quickly find foods that meet your specific needs and goals. According to the FDA, a nutrient content claim on a food product "directly or by implication characterizes the level of a nutrient in a food" (see *www.fda.gov/food/guidanceregulation/guidancedocumentsregulatoryinformation/labelingnutrition/ucm064908.htm*). These claims include terms such as "low-fat," "fat-free," "high in fiber," and "reduced sugar." Each and every claim that is used on a food packaging has a very specific definition governed by the FDA. Here are a few of the more popular ones that are commonly used on food labels.

> ℵ **Reduced or Less:** The food contains at least 25% fewer calories, total fat, saturated fat, sugar, sodium, or cholesterol than the regular product. This might not necessarily mean the product is "low" in the nutrient if the regular product is quite high.

- **Light or Lite:** The food contains one third fewer calories or no more than half the fat of the regular or higher-calorie, higher-fat version, or no more than half the sodium of the higher-sodium version.

- **Good source, Contains, or Provides:** The food contains between 10 and 19 percent of the daily value for a nutrient per serving.

- **Excellent source of, High, Rich in:** The food contains 20 percent or more of the daily value for a nutrient per serving.

- **More, Fortified, Enriched, Added, Extra, or Plus:** The food contains 10 percent or more of the daily value for a nutrient per serving compared to the regular product.

- **No Added Sugars:** No sugar or sugar-containing ingredient is added during processing.

- **Sugar-free:** The food contains less than 0.5 grams of sugar per serving.

- **Low-fat:** The food contains 3 grams of fat or less per serving.

- **Fat-free:** The food contains less than 0.5 grams of fat per serving.

- **Cholesterol-free:** The food contains less than 2 milligrams cholesterol and 2 grams or less of saturated fat per serving.

- **Low-sodium:** The food contains 140 mg or less of sodium per serving.

- ≍ **Sodium-free:** The food contains less than 5 milligrams of sodium per serving.

- ≍ **Low-calorie:** The food contains 40 calories or less per serving.

- ≍ **Calorie-free:** The food contains less than 5 calories per serving.

- ≍ **Lean (on meat labels):** The food contains less than 10 grams of fat per serving, with 4.5 grams or less of saturated fat and 95 milligrams of cholesterol per serving.

- ≍ **Extra Lean (on meat labels):** The food contains less than 5 grams of fat per serving, with less than 2 grams of saturated fat and less than 95 milligrams of cholesterol.

Health Claims on Food labels

Health claims on labels are another tool you can use to help you make healthier choices that are individualized to you and your health issues. The FDA defines a a Health Claim as "any claim made on the label or in labeling of a food, including a dietary supplement, that expressly or by implication, including 'third party' references, written statements, symbols, or vignettes, characterizes the relationship of any substance to a disease or health-related condition. Implied health claims include those statements, symbols, vignettes, or other forms of communication that suggest, within the context in which they are presented, that a relationship exists between the presence or level of a substance in the food and a disease or health-related condition."

Here are examples of just a few health claims:

- ⋊ "Diets rich in whole-grain foods and other plant foods and low in total fat, saturated fat, and cholesterol may help reduce the risk of heart disease."

- ⋊ "Low-fat diets rich in fiber-containing grain products, fruits, and vegetables may reduce the risk of some types of cancer, a disease associated with many factors."

- ⋊ "Low-fat diets rich in fiber-containing grain products, fruits, and vegetables may reduce the risk of some types of cancer, a disease associated with many factors."

To find all of the nutrient content claims and health claims visit the FDA at *www.fda.gov*.

Your Nutrition Solution Tidbit: Need a little more help choosing the right foods? Look for these on food packages as well:

Whole Grains Council Stamp: The **100% stamp** means that all of the grain in the product is whole grain (at least 16 grams of whole grains per serving). The **basic stamp** means the product may contain some extra bran, germ, or refined flour (at least 8 grams of whole grains per serving).

Heart-Check Mark: This means the food product meets the nutrition requirements of the American Heart Association.

chapter 6

14-day menu guide and stocking your kitchen

By now you have learned all you need to know to start using nutrition as your solution to managing acid reflux. This chapter will provide you with 14 days of menus to get you started on the right foot. In addition, this chapter will provide you with an extensive list of all of the foods and beverages that are great to have on hand in your kitchen if you suffer with acid reflux. We know that acid reflux sufferers all have different food triggers, so as you use the tools in this chapter be sure to avoid the foods that may be triggers for you and replace them with foods from your safe list.

14-Day Menu Guide

These menus add up to approximately 2,000 calories per day; you may need to adjust portion sizes depending on your individual calorie intake. All the menus are low in the "bad" fats (saturated and trans fats) and a good source of the "good" fats (the unsaturated fats: polyunsaturated and monounsaturated as well as omega-3 fatty acids). In addition, they are a good source of protein, high in fiber, and high in overall nutritional content. They are approximately 50 percent carbohydrates, 20 percent fats, and 30 percent protein. These menus avoid the common trigger foods we discussed in Chapter 4, and include the foods that may benefit you. The format of these menus follows the recommendation of frequent and smaller meals throughout the day and not eating before bedtime. Adjust the timing of your meals if you work second or third shift and go to bed at an abnormal hour. Drink plenty of water throughout your day.

Day 1

<u>Breakfast</u>

2 cups oatmeal, cooked with water, topped with ½ sliced banana and 5 almonds

1 cup milk, fat-free

Decaf green tea, brewed

A.M. Snack

1 apple, cut in half

1 Tbsp. reduced-fat peanut spread on both halves of apple

6 oz. 100% apple juice

Lunch

Wrap: Chicken salad made with 3 oz. chicken breast, skinless, cooked, and diced; 1 Tbsp. reduced-fat mayonnaise; 1 Tbsp. diced celery. Spread chicken salad on 1 whole-wheat tortilla.

15 grapes, seedless, red or green

½ cup sliced strawberries

P.M. Snack

½ cup low-fat cheddar cheese, cubed

6 whole-wheat reduced-fat crackers

Ginger tea*

Dinner (2–3 hours before bedtime)

6 oz. salmon, wild-caught, grilled or baked (can marinate with teriyaki sauce, Italian dressing, and a few shakes of ground ginger for a few hours before cooking)

8 spears asparagus, fresh, steamed, drizzled with ¼ Tbsp. extra-virgin olive oil

1 cup cooked brown rice mixed with ½ tsp. dried parsley

To make ginger tea: grate about ¼ inch fresh ginger and allow to steep in hot water for about 10 minutes. You can add natural sweetener such as agave nectar or honey.

Day 2

Breakfast

1 English muffin, whole-wheat, toasted, spread with 1 Tbsp. almond butter

2 cups cubed cantaloupe

2 turkey sausage links, cooked

6 oz. fat-free soy milk

Ginger tea

A.M. Snack

6 oz. non-fat Greek yogurt, with 1 Tbsp. ground flaxseed and ½ cup blueberries

Lunch

Sandwich: 4 oz. turkey breast, 2 Tbsp. pureed avocado or guacamole, 2 spinach leaves, on 2 slices whole-wheat bread

8 baby carrots

2 celery stalks, trimmed

2 Tbsp. light ranch dressing for dipping

Chamomile tea, brewed

P.M. Snack

3 rectangle graham cracker squares

20 grapes, seedless, red or green

1 cup fat-free milk

Dinner (2–3 hours before bedtime)

6 oz. skinless chicken breast, baked, broiled, or grilled

1 cup broccoli, steamed

1 medium sweet potato, baked with 1 Tbsp. non-trans-fat margarine

2 cups tossed salad (no tomato or onion) with raw veggies, ¼ cup sliced fennel, ½ Tbsp. extra-virgin olive oil, 1 Tbsp. apple cider vinegar

Day 3

Breakfast

1 ½ cup bran flakes with 1 cup fat-free milk, topped with ½ cup blackberries

1 slice whole-wheat bread, toasted with ½ Tbsp. non-trans-fat margarine

Chamomile tea, brewed

A.M. Snack

1 cup cottage cheese, low-fat

½ cup pineapple chunks, fresh or canned in its own juice

<u>Lunch</u>

2 cups vegetable soup, light

6 whole-wheat crackers

½ cup applesauce, unsweetened

2 celery stalks, trimmed

<u>P.M. Snack</u>

2 rice cakes, brown rice, topped with 1 Tbsp. reduced-fat peanut butter

<u>Dinner (2-3 hours before bedtime)</u>

5 oz. pork chops, boneless, baked, broiled, or grilled

2 cups whole-wheat pasta, cooked and mixed with 1 cup zucchini, steamed, and 1 Tbsp. extra-virgin olive oil

1 cup fat-free milk

Day 4

<u>Breakfast</u>

2 cups oatmeal, cooked with water, topped with ¼ tsp. cinnamon and 10 raisins

½ banana

1 cup fat-free soy milk

Chamomile tea, brewed

<u>A.M. Snack</u>

6 oz. non-fat Greek yogurt with 1 Tbsp. ground flax-seed and ½ cup strawberries, sliced

Lunch

Tuna salad wrap: 3 oz. tuna, canned in water, with 1 Tbsp. reduced-fat mayonnaise, 1 Tbsp. diced celery, and 1 Tbsp. sweet relish. Roll tuna salad in 1 whole-wheat tortilla.

2 cups vegetable soup, light

1 apple

P.M. Snack

½ cup low-fat cheddar cheese, cubed

10 pretzels

6 oz. 100% apple juice

Dinner (2–3 hours before bedtime)

6 oz. flank steak, grilled, baked, or broiled (can sprinkle with ground ginger before cooking and marinade it in your favorite sauce)

1 medium potato, baked and topped with ¼ cup pureed avocado or guacamole

8 spears asparagus, steamed

½ cup carrots, cooked and sprinkled with ¼ Tbsp. dried parsley

Day 5

Breakfast

2 whole-grain waffles, topped with ½ cup blueberries, fresh or frozen, and 2 Tbsp. lite syrup

2 slices turkey bacon, cooked

1 cup milk, fat-free

Ginger tea

A.M. Snack

1 cup cottage cheese, low-fat

1 cup papaya, cubed

Lunch

Sandwich: 3 ounce turkey breast with 1 slice low-fat Swiss cheese, 2 spinach leaves, and 2 Tbsp. pureed avocado or guacamole, on 2 slices whole-wheat bread, toasted

8 baby carrots with 2 Tbsp. light ranch dressing

10 baked tortilla chips

P.M. Snack

1 whole-wheat English muffin, toasted

1 Tbsp. reduced-fat peanut butter

1 cup fat-free milk

Dinner (2–3 hours before bedtime)

Stir-Fry: 5 oz. shrimp, without tails, cut-up; ½ cup fennel, sliced; ½ cup snow peas; ½ cup sweet red peppers; 1 Tbsp. extra-virgin olive oil; 3 Tbsp. soy sauce, light; ½ tsp. ground ginger

Mix all until cooked thoroughly; serve over 1 cup brown rice, cooked

Day 6

Breakfast

2 cups oatmeal, cooked in water, topped with 7 walnut halves and 1 sliced banana

8 oz. fat-free soy milk

Decaf green tea, brewed

A.M. Snack

2 rice cakes, brown rice, topped with 1 Tbsp. almond butter

Ginger tea

Lunch

2 cups salad with fresh veggies (no tomato or onion), topped with 3 oz. canned tuna in water, and ½ Tbsp. extra-virgin olive oil plus 1 Tbsp. apple cider vinegar

6 crackers, whole-wheat

2 cups light soup, chicken, and wild rice with veggies

P.M. Snack

2 rectangle graham crackers

20 grapes, seedless, red or green

<u>Dinner (2–3 hours before bedtime)</u>

Mix together 1 ½ cups pasta, whole-wheat, cooked; ½ cup black beans, canned, drained; ½ cup carrots, steamed; ¼ cup fennel, sliced; ¼ cup peas, steamed; ½ cup zucchini, steamed; ½ Tbsp. extra-virgin olive oil plus 2 Tbsp. freshly grated Parmesan cheese

2 cups salad with raw vegetables (no tomato or onion), topped with ½ Tbsp. extra-virgin olive oil plus 1 Tbsp. apple cider vinegar

Day 7

<u>Breakfast</u>

1 ½ cup bran flakes cereal with ½ cup blueberries and 1 cup fat-free milk

1 slice whole-wheat bread, toasted, topped with ½ Tbsp. non-trans fat margarine

Chamomile tea, brewed

<u>A.M. Snack</u>

6 oz. non-fat Greek yogurt, with 1 Tbsp. ground flaxseed and ½ cup blackberries

<u>Lunch</u>

Sandwich: 4 oz. chicken breast, skinless, sliced; 2 spinach leaves; ¼ cup pureed avocado or guacamole. Wrap in 1 whole-wheat tortilla.

1 cup cucumber slices

10 tortilla chips, baked

Ginger tea

<u>P.M. Snack</u>

1 whole-wheat English muffin, toasted, topped with 1 Tbsp. almond butter

1 apple

<u>Dinner (2–3 hours before bedtime)</u>

6 oz. turkey kielbasa, baked, broiled, or grilled

¾ cup orzo, cooked and mixed with 2 Tbsp. slivered almonds

1 cup broccoli, steamed

> **Your Nutrition Solution Tidbit:** The portion sizes on these menus may not seem important, but you can eat a healthy diet and still eat too much! Portion control is critical to controlling your calorie intake for weight loss and weight maintenance. Don't forget that if your meal gets too big and you stuff yourself you most likely will pay for it with heartburn.

Day 8

<u>Breakfast</u>

4 egg whites scrambled with ¼ cup fresh mushroom and 2 oz. extra-lean diced ham

½ whole-grain bagel topped with ½ Tbsp. non-trans-fat margarine

1 cup strawberries, sliced

Chamomile tea

A.M. Snack

1 cup low-fat cottage cheese

1 cup pineapple chunks, fresh or canned in its own juice

Lunch

2 cups light black-bean soup

6 whole-wheat crackers

1 pear

P.M. Snack

1 banana, spread with 1 Tbsp. reduced-fat peanut butter

1 cup fat-free milk

Dinner (2–3 hours before bedtime)

6 oz. salmon, wild caught, broiled, baked, or grilled (marinate it ahead of time with your favorite sauce such as teriyaki and sprinkle with ginger)

¾ cup wild rice, cooked

½ cup spinach, steamed

1 cup carrots, steamed, with ¼ Tbsp. dried parsley

Day 9

Breakfast

2 cups oatmeal, cooked with water and topped with ½ cup blueberries, ¼ tsp. cinnamon, and 12 raisins

1 cup fat-free milk

Decaf green tea

A.M. Snack

Smoothie: Blend 2 bananas, 1 cup non-fat plain yogurt, 2 cups fat-free soy milk, 2 Tbsp. honey, ½ tsp. ginger root (grated finely), ½ cup ice

Lunch

Wrap: 1 whole-wheat tortilla, 3 slices extra-lean ham, 1 slice low-fat Swiss cheese, ¼ cup diced cucumber, and 1 tsp. yellow mustard

10 tortilla chips, baked

Ginger tea

P.M. Snack

¼ cup hummus with 8 baby carrots

6 whole-wheat crackers

Dinner (2–3 hours before bedtime)

4 oz. Turkey burger, extra lean, grilled or pan-fried

½ whole-wheat pita (6")

1 oz. shredded low fat cheese

¼ cup avocado puree or guacamole

2 spinach leaves

2 cups salad with raw vegetables (no tomato or onion), topped with ½ Tbsp. extra-virgin olive oil plus 1 Tbsp. apple cider vinegar

Day 10

Breakfast

Breakfast sandwich: 4 scrambled egg whites, 1 oz. shredded low-fat cheese, 2 slices Canadian bacon, cooked, all on 1 whole-wheat English muffin, toasted

2 cups diced cantaloupe

1 cup fat-free milk

Chamomile tea

A.M. Snack

6 oz. non-fat Greek yogurt with 1 Tbsp. ground flax-seed and ½ cup fresh raspberries

Lunch

Tuna salad: 3 oz. tuna, canned in water; 1 Tbsp. diced celery; 1 Tbsp. reduced-fat mayonnaise; 1 Tbsp. sweet relish

2 spinach leaves

½ whole-wheat pita (6")

1 cup fat-free milk

1 apple

P.M. Snack

¼ cup pistachios, no shell

5 cups light popcorn, microwave

8 oz. grape juice, red or white

Dinner (2–3 hours before bedtime)

5 oz. flank steak (marinated with your favorite sauce and ground ginger), broiled or grilled

1 medium sweet potato, baked and topped with 1 Tbsp. non-trans-fat margarine and ¼ tsp. cinnamon

1 cup broccoli, steamed

Day 11

Breakfast

Smoothie: Blend 2 bananas, 1 cup non-fat plain yogurt, 2 cups fat-free soy milk, 2 Tbsp. honey, ½ tsp. ginger root (grated finely), ½ cup ice

A.M. Snack

2 rice cakes, brown rice, topped with 1 Tbsp. almond butter

20 grapes, seedless, red or white

Ginger tea

Lunch

Wrap: 4 oz. chicken breast, skinless, cooked, diced; ¼ cup pureed avocado or guacamole; ¼ cup grated carrots; ¼ cup cucumber, diced; 2 spinach leaves; 1 whole-wheat tortilla

12 pretzels

1 pear

P.M. Snack

¼ cup hummus

½ whole-wheat pita (6")

2 celery stalks

Dinner (2–3 hours before bedtime)

6 lean turkey meatballs

1 cup butternut squash, cubed, cooked, topped with 1 Tbsp. non-trans-fat margarine

1 cup steamed green beans

Day 12

Breakfast

1 ½ cups bran flakes with ½ cup fresh raspberries and 1 cup fat-free milk

½ whole-grain bagel topped with 1 Tbsp. reduced-fat peanut butter

Ginger tea

A.M. Snack

1 banana, spread with 1 Tbsp. almond butter

1 cup fat-free milk

Lunch

Sandwich: 2 slices whole-wheat bread, toasted; 3 slices extra-lean ham; 1 slice low-fat Swiss cheese; 2 spinach leaves; ½ Tbsp. reduced-fat mayonnaise

2 cups light vegetable soup

½ cup applesauce, no added sugar

P.M. Snack

1 cup low-fat cottage cheese

1 cup peach slices, fresh or canned in its own juice

Dinner (2–3 hours before bedtime)

6 oz. chicken breast, skinless, baked, broiled, or grilled, topped with 1 Tbsp. teriyaki sauce and ¼ tsp. ground ginger

1 cup brown rice, cooked

1 cup zucchini, steamed

Day 13

Breakfast

2 cups oatmeal, cooked with water and topped with ½ cup raspberries, ¼ tsp. cinnamon, 2 Tbsp. slivered almonds

1 cup fat-free milk

Decaf. Green tea

A.M. Snack

½ cup low-fat cheese, diced

6 whole-wheat crackers

Ginger tea

Lunch

Chicken salad: 3 oz. chicken, breast, skinless, cooked, diced, mixed with 1 Tbsp. diced celery, 1 Tbsp. reduced-fat mayonnaise, 1 Tbsp. sweet relish

½ whole-wheat pita, (6")

1 apple

1 cup fat-free milk

P.M. Snack

¼ cup pistachios, no-shell

5 cups light popcorn, microwave

1 cup grape juice, white or red

Dinner (2–3 hours before bedtime)

5 oz. halibut (marinate with favorite sauce and a sprinkle of ground ginger), baked, broiled, or grilled

1 cup butternut squash, cubed, cooked, topped with 1 Tbsp. non-trans-fat margarine

8 spears asparagus, steamed

Day 14

<u>Breakfast</u>

Breakfast Sandwich: 4 scrambled egg whites; 1 oz. low-fat cheese, shredded; 2 slices Canadian bacon, cooked; all on 1 whole-wheat English muffin, toasted

1 cup strawberries, sliced

1 cup fat-free milk

Chamomile tea

<u>A.M. Snack</u>

6 oz. non-fat Greek yogurt mixed with 1 Tbsp. ground flaxseed, and ½ cup fresh raspberries

<u>Lunch</u>

1 cup low-fat cottage cheese, topped with 1 cup sliced peaches, fresh or canned in its own juice

8 baby carrots

2 celery stalks

Decaf. green tea

<u>P.M. Snack</u>

Smoothie: Blend 2 bananas, 1 cup non-fat plain yogurt 2 cups fat-free soy milk, 2 Tbsp. honey, ½ tsp. ginger root (grated finely) ½ cup ice

<u>Dinner (2–3 hours before bedtime)</u>

6 oz. turkey kielbasa, baked, broiled, or grilled

1 whole-grain hot dog bun

1 tsp. mustard

10 French fries, oven baked

1 cup green beans, steamed

Stocking Your Kitchen

A well-stocked kitchen with plenty of healthy, heartburn-friendly foods will make life much easier. When you know you can grab a healthy snack or a quick meal with the foods you already have in your kitchen, it will relieve some of your stress, which can also be a bonus. You might just find that your whole family will eat healthier once you have your kitchen stocked the right way. This is just sampling of foods to get your started.

Pantry

- Whole-grain bagels, breads, pitas, and wraps
- Instant oatmeal and/or long-cooking oatmeal
- A variety of whole-grain, low-sugar dry cereals
- Brown and/or wild rice
- Quinoa
- Whole-grain couscous
- Whole-grain pasta
- Orzo pasta
- Microwave popcorn, light

- Whole-grain crackers
- Graham crackers
- Rice cakes
- Pretzels
- Baked tortilla chips
- Low-fat granola bars
- A variety of beans, canned or dried (black, navy, red, lima, lentils, chickpeas, soybeans, etc.)
- A variety of light canned soups (avoid those with tomato or are tomato based)
- A variety of canned vegetables with "no salt added" (avoid tomatoes)
- A variety of canned fruit, in water or its own juice (avoid citrus fruits)
- Potatoes, sweet potatoes, and other root vegetables (besides onions)
- Peanut butter
- Nut butters such as almond butter
- Decaf. green tea
- Chamomile tea and other herbal teas
- Apple cider vinegar
- Rice vinegar, flavored
- Extra-virgin olive oil, canola oil, sunflower oil, and/or safflower oil
- Honey
- Ground ginger

- Parsley
- Basil
- Thyme
- Dill
- Onion Powder
- Garlic Powder (many people are bothered by raw garlic so test the waters to see if you do okay with garlic powder)
- Ground cinnamon
- (Any other herb or spice is great to have on hand to add flavor to your meals. Just be aware of which ones cause acid reflux for you.)

Refrigerator

- Milks including fat-free cow's milk, almond milk, and soy milk
- Low-fat cheeses and cottage cheese
- Reduced-fat sour cream
- Non-fat yogurt (Greek yogurt is higher in protein)
- Low-fat puddings (avoid the chocolate varieties)
- Low-fat mayonnaise
- Margarine (trans-fat-free)
- Light salad dressings
- Hummus
- Guacamole

- Fresh veggies including asparagus, beets, bell peppers, endive, carrots, celery, and cucumber
- Dark green leafy veggies such as spinach and kale
- Fennel
- Ginger root
- Green beans
- Mushrooms
- Potatoes, sweet potatoes, and yams
- Salad greens
- Squash such as butternut and zucchini
- Broccoli, cauliflower, and Brussels sprouts
- 100% fruit and vegetable juices (avoid orange, grapefruit, and tomato juices as well as other citrus-based juices)
- Fresh fruit such as apples, apricots (fresh or dried), avocados, berries, melons, peaches, and pears
- Extra-lean ground beef
- Lean cuts of beef (Store meats in the refrigerator for only a few days. It is best to freeze meats and then thaw them for a day or two before using.)
- Skinless poultry
- Lean cuts of pork, fish, and other seafood
- Eggs and egg whites
- Tofu and other soy foods

Freezer

- ✂ Frozen vegetables without sauces
- ✂ Frozen fruits with no added sugar
- ✂ Frozen yogurt and/or low-fat ice cream (avoid chocolate)
- ✂ Sherbet or sorbets
- ✂ Whole-grain waffles, pancakes, French toast
- ✂ Frozen entrees (Look for less than 600 mg sodium, plenty of vegetables, and whole grains. Ensure there are no foods in the meal that are on your avoid list.)

ask the dietitian

We have covered a lot of information in this book, but there are always more questions to be asked and to be answered. Here are a few questions that might just be something you need answered and didn't find it in the book.

Q. How can I find a dietitian that specializes in gastrointestinal disorders such as acid reflux?

A. There are many dietitians out there that provide medical nutrition therapy based on your diagnosis. Many dietitians have their own private practices in which they provide nutrition counseling services, and others provide services through a local clinic or hospital. You can find a dietitian in your area by visiting The Academy of Nutrition and Dietetics (*www.eatright.org*). Include your zip code and/or city and state, the type of service you are looking for, and that you are looking for expertise in digestive disorders and/or gastrointestinal diseases/disorders. You are bound to find one in your area. I have also listed a few dietitians in the resource section of this book that are Certified LEAP Therapists. That would be a good place to start.

Q. Do I need to follow a bland diet if I have acid reflux?

A. I am happy to say that the answer to this question is no. Of course, spicy foods are not the best idea if you are suffering with acid reflux or GERD, but you don't need to follow a bland diet. You can have plenty of taste, fiber, and fresh foods in your diet. Your biggest concern is knowing what your trigger foods are and then staying away from them. Another good reason not to follow a bland diet, which years ago was the go-to diet for those with digestive problems such as GERD, is that some of its recommendations conflict with present dietary recommendations for a healthy eating plan. One of the biggest ones is that bland diets follow a low-fiber intake and we know that fiber is not only part of a healthy diet but it can also be beneficial for people with GERD.

Q. What food would produce acid in the stomach?

A. Foods don't actually produce acid in our stomachs. No food is actually higher in acidity than what our stomach produces. However, any food or beverage that you consume does stimulate the hydrochloric acid that is made by the stomach. So it is your stomach that produces the acid, and certain foods will cause your stomach to produce more acid than others.

Q. Can taking medication for acid reflux/GERD weaken my bones?

A. If your doctor has you on a medication for GERD such as a proton pump inhibitor (PPI), or if you take an over-the-counter version, then yes, you could be at risk for reduced bone health. In 2010 the FDA warned that taking high doses of PPIs for a long period of time could make fractures of the hip, wrist, and spine more likely. The labels of these medications now note that risk. This is another reason you are better off trying to control your acid reflux/GERD with diet and lifestyle changes, and using medication only as a last resort.

Q. I have heard that acid reflux may effect my teeth. How is this possible?

A. People with acid reflux usually feel the burning sensation in the chest area, hence the term "heartburn";

however, not everyone who has GERD has that symptom. Some people have "silent" reflux and don't even realize they have acid reflux. Interestingly, it may be your dentist who actually discovers that there is a problem. The first indication that someone might have GERD is erosion of the enamel on the molars or on the backside of the teeth, caused by stomach acid coming up and actually eating away at the enamel on your teeth. If your dentist detects enamel loss he or she may refer you to a gastroenterologist so that you can be properly diagnosed and treated. Loss of the enamel on your teeth is permanent. If left undetected, it can lead to rapid tooth decay of the affected teeth. Just another important reason to see your dentist regularly and to not let your GERD symptoms go without taking care of them.

Q. Can it be acid reflux that causes my bad breath and the bad taste in my mouth?

A. Yes. The acid that refluxes or flows back up into the esophagus can definitely cause symptoms of bad breath and usually a sour and/or bad taste in the mouth. You can help prevent this by making sure you brush your teeth several times a day, floss on a regular basis, and use mouthwash. You can also chew gum after meals, which can also help with heartburn, but do not choose mint-flavored gum, as mint can have the opposite effect. If you control your acid reflux with diet and lifestyle you will be less likely to deal with this problem.

Q. Are stomach ulcers and heartburn related?

A. Yes, these can be related. Stomach ulcers are sores on the lining of the stomach that occur due to erosion of the stomach lining. That erosion can be caused by GERD. Ulcers can bleed and can cause pain, bloating, and severe heartburn. If you have symptoms of heartburn along with some of these other symptoms you should see your doctor.

Q. Is it possible to get acid reflux or heartburn when your stomach is empty?

A. Yes, it is possible to experience symptoms of acid reflux when your stomach is empty as well as over-full. Both are great reasons to eat small, frequent meals throughout the day. This way you always have something in your stomach but you are never over-stuffing yourself.

Q. Does my age contribute to acid reflux?

A. Unfortunately, as we age we run into a few extra problems. Similar to other muscles in our body, the lower esophageal sphincter (LES) muscle can lose tone and strength as we age. This makes it more likely for the content of our stomach to push up through the weakened valve and cause acid reflux. In addition, the cells in the lining of the stomach can also become less responsive as we age so that the HCL levels naturally decline and complete digestion becomes a bit more difficult. This can also contribute to reflux. To make matter worse for women who are in perimenopause or menopause, hormone replacement therapy has been found to be strongly associated with GERD. Some studies have suggested that elevated levels of estrogen and progesterone, whether they're from our own body or from an outside source such as hormone replacement therapies, can increase symptoms of GERD.

Q. Where can I go for support for GERD?

A. There are plenty of online support groups, forums, and discussion boards available. It is always helpful to have the support of others in your same situation. However, keep in mind that acid reflux and GERD is very individualized, so the fact that one person has certain symptoms and/or triggers does not mean it will be the same for you. That goes for treatment as well. You need to do what you and your doctor feel is best for YOU!

Here are a few sites to get your started:

Healingwell.com
www.healingwell.com/community/?f=45

Med Help
www.medhelp.org/forums/GERD-Acid-Reflux/show/200

WebMd's Heartburn and GERD Community
http://exchanges.webmd.com/gerd-and-heartburn

Health Boards
www.healthboards.com/boards/acid-reflux-gerd/

resources

Websites

About.com:
Heartburn-Free Recipes for the Acid Reflux Diet
http://heartburn.about.com/od/heartburnfreerecipes

American College of Gastroenterology (ACG)
http://gi.org/

The Academy of Nutrition and Dietetics
www.eatright.org

American Gastroenterological Association (AGA)
www.gastro.org

Dietary Guidelines for Americans, 2010
www.health.gov/dietaryguidelines/2010.asp#tools

Dr. Gourmet, GERD-Friendly Recipe Index
www.drgourmet.com/gerd/gerdrecipes.shtml

Esophageal Cancer Action Network:
Reflux Disease (GERD), Barrett's Esophagus and
Esophageal Cancer:
A Guide For Patients
www.ecan.org/site/PageNavigator/Patient_Guide.html

Food Chemicals Codex (FCC)
www.usp.org/food-ingredients/food-chemicals-codex

Health Boards: Acid Reflux/GERD Message Board:
www.healthboards.com/boards/acid-reflux-gerd

Living With Reflux
www.livingwithreflux.org

National Institute of Diabetes and Digestive and Kidney Diseases (NIDDK), National Institutes of Health (NIH):

Gastroesophageal Reflux (GER) and Gastroesophageal Reflux Disease (GERD) in Children and Adolescents

http://digestive.niddk.nih.gov/ddiseases/pubs/ gerinchildren/#symptoms

Pediatric/Adolescent Gastroesophageal Reflux Association

www.reflux.org

RefluxMD

www.refluxmd.com

Teens Health/Gastroesophageal Reflux Disease (GERD)

http://kidshealth.org/teen/diseases_conditions/digestive/gerd. html

U.S. Department of Health and Human Services Physical Activity Guidelines for Americans

www.health.gov/paguidelines

USDA MyPlate.gov

www.choosemyplate.gov

WebMD:
Heartburn/GERD Health Center

www.webmd.com/heartburn-gerd/guide/upper-endoscopy

Certified LEAP Therapists/Dietitians

Oxford Biomedical Technologies

http://nowleap.com/

http://nowleap.com/leap-eating-plan/
leap-anti-inflammatory-eating-plan/

Find a Certified LEAP Therapist: (866) 230-7232

*Many of these Dietitian work via phone and can work with you from an State!

Elizabeth Berry, MS RDN

P: (602) 770-1335

liz@BerryWellCoaching.com

http://BerryWellCoaching.com

www.berrynutrition.com

Facebook: www.facebook.com/berrynutrition.com

Whitney Ahneman, MS, RD, CDN, CLT

White Plains, New York

www.wittynutrition.com

www.maplemedical.com

Susan Linke, MBA, MS, RD, LD, C

Dallas, Texas

www.susanlinke.com

Rita Singer, RD, CLT
Registered Dietitian
Nutrition RS, LLC
Succasunna, New Jersey
P: (862) 239-6370
F: (973) 521-5030
www.nutritionrsllc.com

Amanda Austin, RDN, CLT
Food Sensitivity Specialist
Royal Oak, Michigan
P: (248) 802-8637
E: amanda.austin@getwellified.com
www.getwellified.com

Michaela Ballmann, MS, RD, CLT
Wholify: Restoring Your Wellbeing
Pasadena and Sierra Madre, California
P: (626) 552-9355
www.wholify.com
Twitter: @wholify

Nour Zibdeh, MS, RD, CLT
Nutrition Coach and Owner of Nourition, LLC
Herndon, Virginia

P: (571) 449-6687

E: nour.zibdeh@nourition.com

www.nourition.com

LinkedIn: *www.linkedin.com/in/nourrd*

Facebook: *www.facebook.com/nourition*

Twitter: @NourRD

Alyssa Simpson RD, CDE, CLT

Phoenix, Arizona

P: (480) 703-8883

F: (480) 323-2643

E: Alyssa@nutritionresolution.com

http://nutritionresolution.com/

Sandra Meyerowitz, MPH, RDN, LD

Certified LEAP Therapist

Nutrition Works

Louisville, Kentucky

P: (502) 339-9202

E: sandra@smartnutritionworks.com

www.smartnutritionworks.com

Jan Patenaude, RD, CLT

Director of Medical Nutrition, Oxford Biomedical
Technologies, Inc.

Ft. Collins, Colorado

P: (866) 230-7232

E: DineRight4@aol.com

http://CertifiedLEAPTherapist.com

Facebook: *www.facebook.com/LEAP.MRT*

Twitter: @LEAPMRT

Pinterest: *http://PINTEREST.com/LEAPMRT*

Sharon Richmond, MBA, RD, LDN, CLT

Certificate in Adult Weight Management; Health Coach

Tampa, Florida

P: (813) 727-3219

E: SharonRichmond@nutritionyourweigh.net

www.nutritionyourweigh.net

Jennifer J. Masters, MS, RD, LDN

Certified LEAP Therapist

Pediatric Gastroenterology & Nutritional Support, P.C.

Knoxville, Tennessee

P: (865) 522-4116

www.MyPedsGI.com

Peggy Korody, RD, CLT

Health & Wellness Coach

RD4Health Nutrition Counseling, LLC

Rancho Santa Fe, California

P: (858) 401-9936

E: pkorody@RD4Health.com

www.RD4Health.com

index

about the author

Kimberly A. Tessmer, RDN, LD, is a published au-
thor and consulting dietitian in Brunswick, Ohio. A few of
her most recent books include: *Tell Me what To Eat If I have
Inflammatory Bowel Disease*, *What to Eat If I Am Trying to
Conceive*, *The Complete Idiot's Guide to The Mediterranean
Diet*, and *Tell Me What to Eat If I Have Celiac Disease*.

Kim currently owns and operates Nutrition Focus
(*www.nutrifocus.net*), a consulting company specializing in

weight management, authoring, menu development, and other nutritional services. In addition, Kim acts as the RD on the board of directors for Lifestyles Technologies, Inc., a company that provides nutrition software solutions, developing a wide array of nutritionally sound meal templates.